DELEGATION IN GENERAL PRACTICE

A STUDY OF DOCTORS AND NURSES

DELEGATION IN GENERAL PRACTICE

A STUDY OF DOCTORS AND NURSES

ANN BOWLING

TAVISTOCK PUBLICATIONS

LONDON AND NEW YORK

First published in 1981 by
Tavistock Publications Ltd
11 New Fetter Lane, London EC4P 4EE

Published in the USA by
Tavistock Publications
in association with Methuen, Inc.
733 Third Avenue, New York, NY 10017

© 1981 Ann Bowling

Printed in Great Britain at the
University Press, Cambridge.

British Library Cataloguing in Publication Data

Bowling, Ann
Delegation in general practice.
1. Family medicine
I. Title
362.1'0425   R729.5.G4
ISBN 0–422–77490–1

CONTENTS

CONTENTS

PREFACE

Delegation in General Practice is an analysis of the history of general practice and an investigation of its contemporary problems. It examines the extent to which the delegation of medical tasks to nurses may be a solution to some of these problems and the effect this may have on the development of nursing as a profession.

The description of the history of general practice is included in the first part of this book. It dates from the period when general practitioners were typically known as apothecaries. An awareness of this period is felt to be necessary as it is not possible to understand the current status and attitudes of these doctors without some knowledge of their past. Such an historical analysis reveals the lack of an independent theoretical body of knowledge capable of providing a clear role definition of general practice. This role uncertainty has contributed to the lower status of the general practitioner in relation to the hospital doctor.

Attempts have often been made to develop the role of the general practitioner. It has been suggested that these doctors could concentrate on the emotional problems of patients. Experiments in health education and with various screening techniques suggest they should develop a concern with preventive medicine. Others continue to emphasize the more technical aspects of general medicine. The only role definitions that have become widely accepted are those superficial definitions, usually contained in official reports, describing the general practitioner as professional of first contact, family doctor, personal doctor, and the provider of continuity of care. Discussions of the role of the general practitioner usually neglect the question of whether the suggested roles are legitimate fields of practice, or whether they are merely ideologies representing professional anxieties. This issue is explored by the present author.

One of the factors inhibiting the development of a body of knowledge within general practice may be a lack of experimentation among general practitioners themselves. However, doctors often argue that they do not have the opportunity either to practise or develop their skills because they spend so much time on trivial illness. One method that might allow general practitioners more time to concentrate on developing their skills is the delegation of medical tasks not requiring their level of expertise. Delegation, or the transfer of a task to a person of a lower rank, should be explored. One principal reason is that it is a waste of resources for doctors to perform procedures which others could undertake just as well. This argument is especially powerful in view of the fact that the five-year medical-school training costs approximately £40,000. The case for delegation is valid even in a situation of over-supply of medical manpower as it is still wasteful to expect doctors to perform routine tasks. Moreover, a situation of potential over-supply of doctors is not necessarily going to be the norm in the future, nor does it imply a regional equality in the distribution of doctors. It is also worth considering what is meant by 'over-supply': can supply ever meet demand for health care?

Little research has been carried out on the current extent of the delegation of medical tasks or on its future. The potential for any organizational change depends on the attitudes of affected interest groups towards that change. Again, little is known about the views of health professionals towards delegation. Do doctors want to delegate tasks to non-medical personnel? To whom could they delegate these tasks? Would nurses wish to undertake such a role? How would an expanded nurse role affect nursing as a profession? Such issues are examined in this book and the final chapters analyse them in the context of a survey of the practices and attitudes of sixty-eight randomly selected general practitioners, and seventy-five of their nurses, in four urban areas of England and Wales. Although these cannot be regarded as representative of all general practitioners and nurses working in primary care, there is little reason to believe that they do not represent a reasonable cross-section of such professionals working in urban areas.

One main finding of the present study was that a significant minority of doctors and nurses held unfavourable views towards the delegation of minor clinical tasks and the majority held unfavourable attitudes towards the delegation of diagnostic procedures. General practitioners are in a state of role confusion and it is understandable that a number of them will be reluctant to delegate part of their role.

Nurses are also in a position of role ambiguity and, understandably, may often be reluctant to undertake tasks delegated from another profession. As nursing itself is attempting to achieve professional status, and develop its own independent body of knowledge which would establish its autonomy, the performance of tasks delegated by doctors is not necessarily in its interests. However, as might be expected, treatment room nurses, usually employed by doctors to assist them in their practices, experienced this role confusion less than the district nursing sisters interviewed. The challenge for the future appears to be how to develop an expanded clinical role for nurses in general practice while minimizing role conflict and overlap with doctors, and without conflicting with the professional interests of either group.

Many people made this research project possible. I would like to thank the general practitioners, the district and treatment room nurses who so willingly participated in the study, and the area health authority nursing officers who allowed me to interview their attached nursing staff. I would like to express my gratitude to Professor Roy Mapes who suggested the research topic, and who provided guidance and encouragement during the preparation of the PhD thesis upon which this book is based. I am also grateful to Dr Ann Cartwright, Professor Roy Emerson, Dr David Hall, Dr Barry Reedy, Madeleine Simms, and Dr Gerry Stimson who read and commented on the original version, to Dr Martin Bridgstock and Richard Austin for their assistance with the computer, and to all colleagues at the Medical Sociology Research Centre, Swansea, and at the Institute for Social Studies in Medical Care, London, for their support and encouragement. However, in the final analysis, I must take full responsibility for the views expressed together with any errors or omissions contained in this work. The project was funded by the Social Science Research Council and I am grateful for their financial support. Lastly, I wish to acknowledge the courtesy of the editors of *The Lancet*, *Mims Magazine*, *Nursing Mirror*, *Nursing Times*, and *World Medicine* for allowing me to use previously published material.

ANN BOWLING
October 1980

1

THE DEVELOPMENT OF MEDICINE AS A PROFESSION AND THE EMERGENCE OF THE GENERAL PRACTITIONER

The literature on the subject of the professions and on professionalization is extensive. While there may be a central core of consensus among the theories attempting to answer the question 'What is a profession?', there is also continuing disagreement. What does emerge, however, is the proposition that the professions are those occupations that have successfully prevented the encroachment of rival groups in their particular area of expertise. The possession of autonomy over one's actions is a related factor differentiating professions from other occupations (Freidson 1970). In order to begin to understand the extent to which general practice satisfies the prerequisites of professional status, in particular autonomy of action, the professional status of medicine as a whole requires analysis as well as the process by which it achieved its current position.

During the early period of its existence, medicine was regarded as a trade. Long after the passing of the Middle Ages physicians held little status in society and commanded little respect. However, during the sixteenth and seventeenth centuries medicine gradually became one of the status occupations of the leisured gentry. The latter were a newly emerging group composed of members who did not work in order to be financially reimbursed, but made financial outlays in order to work. They possessed no specialized skills or knowledge, merely an acquaintance with cultural norms. Their social position was dependent upon title, tradition and wealth, not medical expertise. As a result of the limited development of medical knowledge up until 1800, medical practitioners faced much competition from unqualified practitioners, known as quacks. During this period in history, formal medical care was basically provided by three types of practitioner. The first was the physician, who was held to be a

member of a learned profession, and who was responsible for internal
medicine. The second was the surgeon, who was regarded as a
craftsman, and who was responsible for external treatment. Finally,
there was the apothecary, who compounded and dispensed medicines, and who was regarded as a tradesman. In practice, little
difference existed between these groups in terms of the amount of
medical knowledge each possessed. Consequently, patients were
inclined to engage medical practitioners according to their social
status, rather than according to their degree of medical knowledge. In
this respect, the physicians were the élite of the profession. However,
access to formal medical care was limited to a minority of the population, while the less affluent majority relied on informal medical
systems.

The physicians

Attempts were made to control the development of medical services in
England as early as 1421, when interdicts were issued against
unqualified practitioners. In an Act of 1511, Henry VIII stated that
the physicians and surgeons in every diocese must be licensed by the
bishop. Prior to 1511 the physicians possessed no monopolistic rights.
Apothecaries and surgeons were permitted to dispense advice as well
as goods and services without infringing the legal rights of the
physicians, although they did trespass upon the physician's preserve.
Nor did the former two groups encroach upon the guild rights of the
latter, as the physicians were not regarded as a guild. Although the
1511 Act aimed at restricting the practice of medicine to those who
had been examined by the ecclesiastical authorities, no administrative apparatus was established to implement this statute. The
physicians' solution was to establish the Royal College of Physicians
in 1518, in the hope that the formation of a prestigious body would
help them make a monopolistic claim on the provision of medical
care. They were assisted in the formation of the College by Henry
VIII himself, whose fear of illness and of being treated by unqualified
practitioners was aggravated by an outbreak of plague. The establishment of the College (which took place despite the limited amount
of knowledge possessed by even those who were qualified) was the
first instance of the licensing of physicians by a purely professional
body, rather than by the Church, the State, or the universities.

It was also the first example of the modern concept of the medical
profession as a body of self-regulating practitioners who assume
authority on the basis of their claim to knowledge. However, the

physicians still faced the possibility of the king removing their Royal Charter should they fall into disfavour. This was a realistic possibility whilst medical science was still at an embryonic stage. Consequently, the College turned to Parliament in 1523 for an Act to secure its Charter under statutory law, attempting to legitimize its existence by associating itself with the concept of a national service. By doing so, it distinguished itself not only from the trades and crafts but also from the surgeons and apothecaries. However, internal quarrels existed within the College. The élite of the College were the Fellows, who were graduates of Oxbridge. The second tier was composed of the Licentiates who, unlike the Fellows, held no political offices or decision-making positions and could practise only within a seven-mile radius of London. Inevitably, relationships between the Fellows and the Licentiates were bitter. Despite such feelings of conflict, the modern concept of a profession had begun to emerge. The physicians' monopolistic privileges were guaranteed legislatively and in future their professional aims and actions were to be determined only by physicians.

The physicians were not only regarded as the élite sector of all medical practitioners, but also as the social and educational superiors of the surgeons and apothecaries. By 1800, physicians came from the more prosperous middle-class section of society. They were the sons of physicians themselves, of the more affluent members of the clergy, of lawyers and other professional families, and some were members of the upper classes. Their education was superior to that of the other two types of medical practitioner in a cultural rather than in a medical sense. Many physicians received only one year's training in medical knowledge and the student was left to decide upon his own medical curriculum and the best methods of assimilating it.

Medical education in Scotland was different. It was organized by the universities with the result that in the eighteenth century Scotland possessed the best medical schools in Europe. Over a period of three years, medical students in Scotland attended courses in anatomy, surgery, pharmacy, the theory and practice of medicine, clinical medicine, midwifery, chemistry and botany, amongst others. In addition, they had to complete a three-month course in two of the following subjects: practical anatomy, natural history, medical juris-prudence, clinical surgery, and military surgery. With such an advanced degree of organization it is perhaps surprising that London physicians were so highly regarded. However, the concern of the Royal College of Physicians to retain its privileges and maintain the distinctions between the various types of medical practitioners may be seen as an example of an emerging organization whose main interest appeared to be the status of the profession itself. Although professional organizations justify their existence by claiming to control unlawful or dangerous practice in the interests of the consumer, it is also in their own interests to do so. Such control leads to their own position of professional monopoly and autonomy.

The surgeons

In the eighteenth century the surgeons were not scholars but craftsmen, organized in a guild which was associated with the barbers until 1745. They were licensed to perform procedures which could be carried out on unanaesthetized patients and until 1700 treatment generally took place in the patient's home. Between 1700 and 1850 this situation altered due to the rise of the voluntary hospitals which provided a setting for developments in surgery. As a result, the prestige of the surgeons gradually rose and enabled them to break away from the barbers in 1745 with the foundation of the Company of Surgeons. However, no body of knowledge on which to base surgery had as yet been formulated. In theory, there was a clear distinction between surgery and physic: surgery was regarded as crude, physic as an art. Although prescribing was the domain of the physician, the surgeon would prescribe if necessary and thus, in practice, the distinction was less clear. There was a crucial difference between these two types of practitioner in a further sense – the physicians attracted patients of great affluence while the less affluent turned to the surgeons for medical advice. Of course, the lower social classes could rarely afford to employ the services of any formal medical practitioner. Home remedies and lay advice were their source of health care, and only in the last resort was treatment received from a Charity or Poor Law Hospital.

No professional organization existed for the surgeon in the eighteenth century; nor were there any legal requirements enforcing an education. Although the educational backgrounds of the physicians and surgeons differed considerably, there is less certainty concerning the social origins of the surgeons. It is possible that they came from a similar background to the physicians, but included slightly less affluent individuals, as the training for surgery was less expensive. The increasing status of the surgeons enabled them to establish their own Royal College in 1800. They achieved this with the assistance of the Royal College of Physicians, who simultaneously managed to reinforce the distinctions between the two groups. Educational requirements were not notably more stringent after the establishment of the Royal College of Surgeons. The London College's educational requirements for their examination had merely consisted of certificates of one course in anatomy and one in surgery but in 1813 the College voluntarily included one year's attendance at the surgical practice of a hospital. Attendance at operations was also compulsory. However, until further advances in surgery were made, the physicians remained the élite professional medical body.

The apothecaries

The apothecaries were initially recognized in 1543 as a result of an Act that acknowledged the skills of lay people with a knowledge of the medical use of herbal remedies. They worked with their hands, performing the more practical aspects of medicine such as cupping and bleeding, and were primarily shopkeepers, selling drugs – hence the label of tradesmen.

The apothecary, like the general practitioner who emerged later, had the lowest social status of all the medical orders, and possessed no learned body of knowledge. Apothecaries came from families of shopkeepers and other lower middle-class groups. Their education was practical and their training was that of other mercantile trades: apprenticeship. They were the largest group of recognized medical practitioners and experienced direct competition from unqualified practitioners. The chemists and druggists, who initially passed drugs from importers to the apothecaries, were also retailing their remedies direct to the public by the eighteenth century, thus acting in direct competition to the apothecaries. The latter group responded by becoming more involved in visiting and treating the sick as well as in the prescribing of drugs, thereby infringing upon the physicians' role. The apothecaries were in an increasingly unfortunate position: the lowest social-status group within the formal medical hierarchy, they received the least respect from the general public, and were regarded with disdain both by physicians and surgeons. Even the surgeons would not admit anyone who practised pharmacy to their Fellowship. The contempt felt by the physicians for the apothecaries was heightened by the latter's increasing tendency to prescribe for people they visited and for anyone who entered their shops.

One way in which the Royal College of Physicians attempted to eliminate its competitors was by helping the apothecaries to create their own guild in 1614. The use of their influence to assist the weak faction of apothecaries to break away from the Grocers' Company seemed to be within the physicians' interests. One of the terms of agreement between the apothecaries, the grocers, and the physicians was that the apothecaries should not make up prescriptions other than those of the physicians recognized by the Royal College. Thus, in 1617 the apothecaries were incorporated as a company and were royally proclaimed in 1620. After 1684 their company was known as the Society of Apothecaries. However, the physicians' scheme failed. As the College did nothing to attempt to eliminate illegal practitioners, the apothecaries felt that it did not support its monopolistic claims under the guild system. Many apothecaries also regarded the privileges of the physicians as unjustified. Together with the surgeons, they felt that since most of the medical practitioners in England were not physicians, equal licensing privileges should be extended to all groups. Surgeons and apothecaries both wished to share the prestige emanating from the concept of the profession created by the Royal College of Physicians.

The apothecaries eventually acquired the right to diagnose and treat the sick during the plague of 1665, when the upper classes left London, soon to be followed by the physicians – who were pursuing their income and their safety. From this time on the apothecaries extended their medical functions in spite of the physicians' attempts to re-establish their monopoly by legal action in 1703. However, the House of Lords upheld the apothecaries' rights to see patients and prescribe medicines. This became a standing grievance with the physicians, who argued that the apothecaries lived not by charging for attendance and advice, in a professional manner, but by selling drugs, like tradesmen. This gave them a direct interest in the quantity of drugs sold and was not professionally ethical. In 1834 most witnesses before the Select Committee enquiring into the case agreed that this practice should cease. It was felt that the apothecaries should charge for attendance and leave the drug industry to the chemists and druggists. The problem for the apothecaries was that the attendance charge did not yield them sufficient income, and if this fee was increased many people would not be able to afford it. On the other hand, the apothecaries disliked the similarity of their trade to that of the chemists and druggists, as they rated themselves superior to these groups. In practice, the only difference between them was that the chemists and druggists were shop-bound. The manoeuvre suggested by the Select Committee was therefore appealing as it would enable the apothecaries to clarify the distinction between themselves and these two groups. The chemists and druggists fought against being cut off from the medical profession, but in 1841 they acknowledged defeat by establishing their own professional body, the Pharmaceutical Society.

Because of the gradual accumulation of power by the apothecaries and surgeons, the Royal College of Physicians decided to adopt the strategy of supporting the movement for licensing privileges among these two groups, but to reject equal privileges. By the end of the eighteenth century the Royal College of Physicians agreed to admit both the surgeons and the apothecaries to the medical profession, on the condition that the unique position of the physicians be maintained. Consequently, the surgeons received their Royal Charter for a Royal College of Surgeons in 1797 at the suggestion of the physicians, and the Royal College of Surgeons was eventually established in 1800. Unlike the Royal College of Physicians, the Royal College of Surgeons had no coercive powers. It merely had the function of conducting examinations and issuing licences. More than the surgeons, it was the apothecaries who had usurped the physicians' role. Thus, when the Society of Apothecaries was converted into an examining body in 1815, the physicians supported the move because the former set lower standards for their licence, hence preserving the physicians' higher prestige. Each step the apothecaries took towards becoming a member of the medical profession was at the expense of accepting a lower status than the dominant groups. This was a pattern to be repeated throughout the history of the apothecary and later of the general practitioner. It is a typical pattern in the development of the professions whereby professional bodies aim to exclude competitors or control them.

The Apothecaries' Act of 1815

It was the apothecaries who first established a modern system of qualification and registration. Their aim was to increase their status, to end the competition from unqualified practitioners, to secure self-government, and to terminate the overall authority of the physicians. Their success was initially marked by the Apothecaries' Act passed in 1815. This gave them the power to determine the educational requirements for entry into their profession, to examine for proficiency, and, on the basis of examination results, to grant or withhold licences which, alone, would authorize their holders to call themselves apothecaries. The Act also gave the Society the power to prevent unqualified persons calling themselves apothecaries in England and Wales. The effect was to provide a secure basis for the licensing and regulation of medicine at the level of the apothecary. All apothecaries, and in effect all practitioners of general medicine in the future, would have to be examined and licensed by the Society of Apothecaries. Moreover, the student was compelled to complete at least five years of apprenticeship before the examination could take place. The powers granted to the apothecaries exceeded those granted to the physicians and surgeons, for although both Royal Colleges were examining bodies, the surgeons possessed no powers to prevent anyone adopting the title of surgeon, and the authority of the physicians extended only to within a seven-mile radius of London.

Although the Royal College of Physicians had supported the 1815 Act to the extent that it preserved their own higher prestige and vested interests, both Royal Colleges remained aloof from the problems experienced by the apothecaries. The physicians and surgeons had a higher social status than the apothecaries and were determined to retain it. They had no wish to include the apothecaries within their membership and risk a lowering of their status. However, the division between the three groups was less distinct than the two Royal Colleges maintained, as many apothecaries possessed licensure of the Society of Apothecaries as well as membership of the Royal College of Surgeons. Resistance on the part of the Royal Colleges may have been partly responsible for the apothecaries' success in persuading the Government to pass the 1815 Act.

The Act itself was not passed without conflict among the medical orders. The movement which led to the passing of the legislation began in 1804 when the Royal College of Physicians and the Lincolnshire Benevolent Medical Society, a provincial general practitioners' organization, began to consider measures to restrain unqualified practitioners. A leading figure in the movement on the Lincolnshire side, Dr Edward Harrison, developed a friendly relationship with the Master of the Royal College of Surgeons and with the President of the Royal College of Physicians. As a result, they formed a body called the Associated Faculty to campaign for the required legislation. However, the Royal College of Physicians had no wish to co-operate on equal terms with the surgeons or the apothecaries. The surgeons, too, on at least one occasion caused the Act to be withdrawn. The chemists and druggists also opposed the movement because they felt it would depress their status and suppress their chances of enhancing it in the future. The campaign for the Act developed into yet another political conflict which was to repeat itself in the movement towards the Medical Act of 1858.

In its final form, the 1815 Act has been variously regarded as a remarkable achievement for the apothecaries and as a disaster

(Newman 1957; Holloway 1966). On the one hand, it could be argued that the only organization to benefit from the Act was the Royal College of Physicians. The physicians had not opposed the Act because they were afraid that if they did not participate the reformers would achieve their objectives in spite of them. By participating, they could attempt to safeguard their higher status. The Act reflected this by placing the Society of Apothecaries under the guardianship of the Royal College of Physicians. For example, the physicians had insisted that the Act should make it an offence for the apothecaries to refuse to compound the physicians' prescriptions. The Act also emphasized the low status of the apothecaries by stressing their guild and trading activities. The retail aspect of their work was reinforced by the insistence upon the retention of a five-year apprenticeship, an extremely controversial clause as apprenticeship was the qualification honoured by trades and crafts. The clause that all general practitioners were legally required to pass the examination of the Society of Apothecaries after experiencing a five-year apprenticeship led to much dissatisfaction. Practitioners, other than apothecaries, felt resentment that the lowly body of apothecaries could suddenly be invested with the power to regulate general medical practice. The Scottish-trained physicians were particularly displeased by the apprenticeship clause as they had already experienced a medical education of high standard. The physicians had also insisted that the Act should state that apothecaries could no longer charge for advice. Instead they had to rely on guild-like income from medications. Finally, the Act did not restrict the practice of the druggists and chemists, the apothecaries' main competitors, a reflection of the pressure these two groups had exerted on the House of Commons.

However, not all the controversial aspects of the Act remained. The chemists and druggists were eventually prevented from prescribing medicines and selling self-prescribed remedies in their shops. The apprenticeship system was also eventually superseded by a curriculum of medical education. Furthermore, a court decision of 1811 had permitted fees for advice from apothecaries, and subsequent court decisions did not uphold the conditions relating to charges under the 1815 Act. By 1829 apothecaries could legally choose to charge for attendances. The Act also had a number of beneficial effects. For example, it was the apothecaries who, through the 1815 Act, pioneered improvements in the standard of medical education, thereby raising the status of the medical profession. A week after the Act was passed the apothecaries had set up a Court of Examiners. The Court's regulations for a professional education included a knowledge of Latin, certificates of attendance at lectures on anatomy, physiology, medicine, chemistry, and therapeutics, in addition to six months' hospital attendance and five years' apprenticeship. The apothecaries insisted upon formal examinations, not mere interviews as at Oxford and Cambridge, and consequently their educational system acquired considerable prestige. The surgeons soon followed their example and upgraded their own educational requirements and examinations.

Although the physicians still retained their élite position in a now extended medical world, the Act was an important landmark in the history of the development of medicine as a profession. Before the medical profession could be identified as a legitimate group of experts by the state it first had to establish its public identity and visibility. Stringent examinations leading to recognizable qualifications was an essential prerequisite of this legitimacy. In fact, the 1815 Act provided a model for the development of a profession. It demonstrated that an organization may become self-governing, it gave statutory force to the notion of formal professional education under the control of a professional body, and tested potential apothecaries by strict examination. The standing and independence of the professional body was emphasized by the licensing power given to the Society of Apothecaries. Finally, it made unqualified medical practice more difficult and created a precedent for future legislation.

The Medical Act of 1858

The position of the apothecary was further improved by the Medical Act of 1858 which resulted in a unification of the profession and created an official council, the General Council of Medical Education and Registration, now the General Medical Council. The 1858 Act was the seventeenth in a series of bills presented to Parliament from 1840 onwards and was the result of an awareness of the newly emerging conception of a profession as a unified and self-governing body. The many unsuccessful attempts to introduce the Act, however, reflected the lack of solidarity within the medical profession and, ironically, the opposition of two of the medical hierarchies to the concept of a united profession in which all practitioners would have equal status before the law. The Royal College of Physicians and the Royal College of Surgeons were already powerful bodies and felt they had little to gain from an Act which gave the lower ranks status equal to their own.

The main advantage of the Act was that it created the registered medical practitioner who was compelled to satisfy one or more of the twenty-one existing licensing bodies, after examination, that s/he was fit to practise. The powers of the existing licensing bodies now covered the United Kingdom, instead of being confined to certain areas. A licence granted by such a body gave holders the right to have their names placed on the register of the newly created General Council of Medical Education and Registration. Not only could registered doctors practise anywhere in the United Kingdom, but they could also practise any branch of medicine.

The purpose of the new Council was to regulate the standards of examining bodies; consequently it was empowered to remove practitioners from the register under certain circumstances and to refuse to accept licences from corporations not meeting minimal examination standards. It did not legally restrict practice to members of the interest group, it did not exercise sole control over entry into the group, and it did not prosecute competitors. The Council, however, became the central body for disciplining the whole profession. Moreover, although the Crown and the universities also wielded power in the appointment of its members, nine out of the twenty-three members of the Council were appointed by the medical corporations, these nine being the largest single group on the Council. The establishment and composition of the Council appeared to confirm the concept that the professions should be responsible for their own conduct. It was unfortunate for the medical profession that the concept of monopoly of practice was not also fulfilled. Parliament, with its liberal policy of inaction, refused to outlaw unqualified practitioners; it merely placed them at a disadvantage by refusing to allow them to sign statutory certificates or prescribe dangerous drugs. An unregistered person who performed a surgical operation could be charged with assault and possibly with manslaughter. After 1858, only a registered medical practitioner could hold an official appointment, for example in a hospital. The Act also finally excluded the chemists and druggists from the medical profession. Together with the 1815 Apothecaries' Act, the 1858 Medical Act became one of the forerunners of improvements in medical education.

Once established, the Council felt that if a unified profession was to be realized, it would require efforts at homogenization based on a standard level of education. The desirable preliminary education for medicine increasingly became the public school. In 1859 the first Committee on Education established by the Council stated that members of the medical profession should have received an education in general knowledge equal to that required by the universities.

Apprenticeships, which were already declining, were further affected by this educational philosophy. Over the years they had gradually become combined with attendance at lectures and practical experience in a recognized hospital medical school. This combination was made compulsory as a condition of qualification by the Apothecaries' Hall. In 1874 an Act allowed the requirements of apprenticeship to be bypassed, and in 1907 the Society of Apothecaries was empowered to give a complete medical qualification.

Although the 1858 Act enhanced the power of the apothecaries by including them in a unified medical profession, it did little to alter the overall balance of power. The pre-eminence and influence of the Royal College of Physicians remained intact. There was little representation for the vast majority of general practitioners, apart from two apothecaries' organizations on the Council. Presumably, the government felt reluctant to offend such a traditionally powerful organization as the Royal College of Physicians, which was closely related to the establishment and élite sections of society. However, the Medical Registration Act of 1858 was still a major landmark in the rise of the apothecary and the surgeon from their lowly status of tradesman and craftsman and their assimilation into a unified medical profession with the higher status physicians.

What led to the development of an autonomous medical profession in a period when medicine could not yet intervene effectively in illness? Medicine established its monopoly position at this time only partly because of patronage from the ruling classes. Certainly, élite groups do demonstrate solidarity with each other. However, one main factor was the rapidly expanding middle class, a product of the Industrial Revolution, who, with their rising expectations of health care, provided a new clientele for doctors. The 1858 Act was also passed because the lower ranks of the profession, the apothecaries, had achieved sufficient unity to possess real power and to occupy an effective bargaining position within the profession. Their relative influence was growing due to the emerging solidarity between themselves and the fourth expanding branch of the profession, the Poor Law medical officers, as a result of their common desire to receive protection from unlicensed practitioners. This shared interest eventually overcame the élitism of the Royal Colleges.

Perhaps the most important reason why the Act was passed at this time was the spirit of reform sweeping through the early nineteenth century. The Industrial Revolution brought about a considerable growth of the middle and working classes and increased their political power. The consequence was that both classes united to counteract the dominant position of the upper classes. This unification and demand for reform found expression in the political representatives of the middle class, the Liberal party, which controlled the government at that time. The 1832 Reform Bill had succeeded in eradicating the old rotten boroughs, thus removing some of the corruption from the selection process for membership of the House of Commons. The retention of power and privilege by the élite members of the profession was incompatible with this climate of opinion and the way was paved for government reform within the medical profession.

The year 1858, then, saw the establishment of Freidson's first two conditions for the emergence of functional autonomy for the medical profession (Freidson 1970). These were a system of registration and licensing for medical practitioners, and the essential first steps towards enabling the profession to control the recruitment and training of its members. The professions are very much a Victorian creation and by 1860 the essential elements of professional status were clear. Reader (1966) has illustrated that they consisted of the formation of a professional association to express the opinions of the profession, to create a body of knowledge, and to regulate codes of conduct. It was also held that a profession should possess a Royal Charter and that Parliament should pass an Act conferring monopoly powers on its qualified practitioners. Other occupations followed the example of medicine in its method of achieving professional status throughout the rest of the nineteenth century and into the twentieth century.

The development of the referral system

With the later introduction of aseptic techniques, and anaesthetics, and the development of the germ theory of disease, the status of medicine, particularly of surgery, increased. During the second half of the nineteenth century, surgeons and physicians began to control the voluntary hospitals and the emerging specialist hospitals, laying the foundations for their dominance within the medical hierarchy as the custodians of specialist knowledge. With the development of more sophisticated medical knowledge the hospitals became increasingly attractive to the middle and upper classes seeking medical care. By the last quarter of the nineteenth century the new specialist hospitals were increasingly being used to treat the minor medical conditions of middle-class patients. The voluntary hospital had traditionally offered medical treatment to the seriously ill poor. However, the expansion of teaching in these hospitals led to an increase in the treatment of poorer people in out-patient departments. Hospital doctors were reluctant to use their private patients as teaching material for their students. Consequently, the general practitioners, as apothecaries were gradually becoming called after 1815, were threatened with the loss of patients from both ends of the social scale. The loss of middle-class patients threatened both their income and their status, for by becoming doctors for the middle classes, general practitioners had hoped to see their profession identified with the status of gentleman. The loss of patients to the hospitals also occurred at a time when they were attempting to establish themselves as doctors of first contact. Their position was once again threatened.

Hospital doctors were reluctant to re-divert middle-class patients to general practitioners, as the tradition of unpaid service for hospital doctors still prevailed. They relied for their livelihood upon income from private practice tending the more affluent classes. In 1886 general practitioners formed the Association of General Practitioners, an offshoot of the British Medical Association, with the aim of forcing specialists to confine their activities to hospital practice and consulting. In June, 1886 a circular was reproduced in the *British Medical Journal*, appealing for support for the Association and suggesting that the general practitioner should apply to the consultant on behalf of the patient where referral to a specialist was necessary. Gradually, the principle of referral became accepted. Primary care became the exclusive domain of the general practitioner and, with few exceptions, patients could gain access to hospital specialists only through general practitioners. However, this improved power position and remuneration were not to last and general practitioners once more found themselves at a disadvantage as hospital medicine, from which they were now largely excluded, became more scientific and thus more prestigious. The establishment of the referral system laid the foundations for the future. Hospital medicine would continue to become prestigious and hospital doctors would benefit from high income and social standing. General practice, on the other hand, gradually became regarded as unstimulating and suitable only for those who had fallen off the ladder of success in their hospital careers (Moran 1958). The hospital, and hence the physicians and surgeons, was once again threatening the position and status of the general practitioner. Moreover, medical education was also being taken over by the hospitals as apprenticeship to an apothecary became replaced by a hospital medical school training. Where hospital practice was concerned, it was only in the rural areas, with the existence of the cottage hospitals, that the general practitioner continued to play a role in hospital life.

The Health Insurance Act of 1911

Freidson's (1970) third condition for the establishment of professional autonomy is public belief in the occupation's competence, and in the values of its knowledge and skill. The emergence of this final condition is difficult to locate in the history of the medical profession. The exclusiveness of medicine is still not totally assured as people continue to resort to self-treatment as well as to unorthodox healers. However, in 1911 the Health Insurance Act was passed. This ensured primary medical care for the working sector of the population and recognized the medical profession as the providers of this care.

The growth of the working classes and the trade union movement strengthened the campaign for health insurance. An increasing militancy, resulting in a high number of strikes during the early 1900s throughout Europe, was initiated by the Soviet Revolution of 1905. The working population began to demand higher wages, improved working conditions, and job security. The ruling classes were forced to meet such demands in order to maintain productivity. The need for improved health care facilities for the working classes was recognized because of the problem of sickness absenteeism which resulted in reduced productivity. The poor health of workers was increasingly evident and vast numbers were rejected on medical grounds as soldiers for the Boer War (Navarro 1978). In the health sector, then, the concession made to this less affluent section of society was the Insurance Act of 1911.

The 1911 Act, modelled upon Bismark's legislation in Germany, insured workers, but not their dependants, against illness and made financial provision for their treatment. Workers who earned less than £160 per annum were to pay four pence each week into the Insurance Fund, while for each insured worker the employer was to contribute three pence and the Treasury two pence. In return, the guaranteed benefit was ten shillings a week in cases of sickness and free medical attention from doctors participating in the 'panel system'. The panel was the list of insured patients doctors became responsible for; this was in addition to any private patients they might treat. The provisions of the Act did not cover the cost of specialist services, hospital, dental, or ophthalmic treatment.

The Act did not represent initial government recognition of the medical profession; the 1858 Act had done this. Berlant (1975) has argued that earlier State involvement in the profession's affairs represented a solution to the failure of the profession adequately to eliminate competitors. For example, throughout its history the Royal College of Physicians had surrendered certain monopolistic privileges in exchange for the introduction of deterrents to unqualified practice. The 1911 Act was one such deterrent, representing State recognition of the medical profession. It was an Act that gave wider recognition to the medical profession than had previous Acts. Moreover, it was an Act which was made possible only by the previous Act of 1858, which had created a unified profession.

What effect did the 1911 Act have upon the functional autonomy of the profession? Although the Act, by virtue of the 'panel system', improved the financial position of general practitioners, it did introduce a degree of State regulation. The initial formulation of the Bill had placed the control of the medical benefit in the hands of the friendly societies, who had previously organized private health insurance. In addition, it had not allowed for free choice of doctor, and it had not given the medical profession representation on administrative committees. The British Medical Association recognized the potential threat to doctors' autonomy and, in confrontations with the Government, demanded six cardinal concessions in June, 1911. These points consisted of an income limit of two pounds a week for those receiving medical benefit, free choice of doctor by patient with the agreement of the doctor to treat the patient, medical and maternity benefits to be administered by the proposed health committees instead of by the friendly societies, the method of doctors' remuneration to be fixed according to the majority of the medical profession on each health committee's district, medical remuneration to be fixed at a level which the profession considered adequate, and adequate representation of the medical profession on the central and local administrative bodies which were being set up to administer the scheme.

Four of these six points were incorporated into the Act. The Government refused to accept the first point, and debate continued on the issue of doctors' remuneration. Despite the threat of resignation and non-cooperation by the medical profession, the Act was passed in the autumn of 1911. The medical profession had nevertheless emerged as a powerful pressure group which could insist upon conditions of practice in its negotiations with the Government, and the achievement of four of the six points had enhanced its functional autonomy. It was also advantageous to the profession and the public that doctors could now treat their poorer patients without reference to their ability to pay for the treatment. This enhanced doctors' clinical autonomy, since they could now undertake treatment according to the current state of medical knowledge rather than according to patients' financial circumstances. On the other hand, one disadvantage was that the more expensive the treatment or prescription issued, the lower the doctor's income. It became financially advantageous to refer patients requiring expensive care to a hospital out-patient department.

Overall, under the Act medical practitioners undoubtedly secured a strengthening of self-government. In order to protect the panel practitioner from unfair treatment by local insurance committees, doctors were given considerable scope to participate in the administration of the Act. The Act provided for a local medical committee elected by medical practitioners and representatives of those members of the profession who accepted service under the Act. These committees were empowered to investigate and report on all complaints made by one practitioner against another, questions concerning clinical conduct and treatment, and complaints of extravagant prescribing and other malpractices by panel practitioners. The insurance commissioners in the United Kingdom also included one medical practitioner appointed by the Government. Medical representation was strengthened when administration of the scheme was passed to the Ministry of Health, created in 1919. Representation was then located in the Central Advisory Committee.

On the other hand, a degree of State regulation of the profession was imposed. Although medical practitioners were now entitled to be on the 'panel' for their district and to receive a capitation fee for each person on their list, they had to provide adequate treatment as defined by the Act. They were required to complete certain forms, make returns to the local insurance committees, and provide certificates of incapacity for work. The approved societies were empowered to send their own medical practitioners to visit the patient to give second opinions of the patient's condition. The cost of prescriptions was liable to be scrutinized and, if thought to be extravagant, the doctor could be surcharged. The freedom of the doctor and the patient to negotiate treatment and payment was eliminated under this scheme. However, despite the threat of government interference, medical practitioners strengthened their autonomy in so far as they achieved a greater degree of self-government. Not only did the 1911 Act further the process of professionalization in medicine, but it also reinforced the position of the general medical practitioner. It substantially increased the income of these doctors, led to an increase in their number and brought the mass of the working population into contact with them. By doing so, it established the concept of the family doctor and reinforced the referral system. General practice was thus given support at a time when it was being seriously threatened by hospital practice.

The National Health Service Act of 1946

As a result of increasing unrest among the working classes, further aggravated by the Wall Street crash of 1929 signalling world depression, the Labour Party increased its demands for a more complete medical service for the population. Although plans were postponed with the beginning of the Second World War, the end of the war renewed class antagonisms and demands within the Labour Party for social change. In the health sector the response to increasing unrest was the passing of the National Health Service Act of 1946. The form the Act took, however, was influenced by professional pressure groups. For example, it enhanced the power of the medical profession, despite the latter's fears of greater State regulation. From the newly created Central Health Services Council downwards there was substantial medical representation. The rights of part-time service and of private practice were retained. With the introduction of the distinction awards system for hospital doctors, large sums of public money were allocated by consultants to other outstanding consultants. Bevan made such concessions to ensure the co-operation of the medical profession, as without it a National Health Service would not have been possible. Furthermore, committees for appointing hospital consultants consisted of at least five doctors out of a total of seven members. Review committees to assess and grade hospital staff were composed entirely of specialists. General practitioners maintained their position as independent contractors who could withdraw from the Service if they regarded their contracts as inadequate.

What effect did the Act have on the status of the general practitioner? These doctors gained a more secure position, a higher rate of remuneration, and a narrowing of the social gap between general practitioners and hospital doctors. However, their differential bargaining power remained. This ensured that, in their debates with the Government prior to the passing of the Act, hospital doctors would achieve most of their demands while the less powerful generalists, together with the public health practitioners, would not. Moreover, before 1948 when the National Health Service was inaugurated, the consultant was still dependent on the goodwill of the general practitioner for the referral of private patients.

Once the National Health Service Act had given the consultants their financial independence, they were free to regard generalists with the derision that stemmed from an era which valued specialism. The specialists had the further advantage of a salary with favourable scales of remuneration. A salaried service had been rejected by general practitioners on the grounds that it would interfere with their independence. The specialists' prejudices against such a system were overcome by the creation of regional hospital boards – now known as regional health authorities – with whom they could have a contractual relationship. The financial position of the specialists was also more advantageous than that of the general practitioners. They were awarded paid holidays, a benefit general practitioners did not achieve until later on; they did not have to employ locums to cover their off-duty periods; they had study leave, free secretarial and ancillary help, and a generous pension plan.

In contrast, there was little financial incentive for general practitioners to practise an adequate standard of care. Because of the capitation system which they had chosen, their remuneration was the same regardless of the amount of time and energy they spent on their practices. As they were, and still are, remunerated according to the number of patients on their lists, it was financially rewarding to possess a high list and perform as few services as possible for the patients. In addition, by acceding to the requests of the hospital doctors, or specialists, the Government could utilize the 'élite's' agreement to its plans in its negotiations with the general practitioners. It thus became increasingly difficult for general practitioners to argue in favour of retaining such rights as the buying and selling of practices. Their bargaining position was further undermined by their lack of a clear role definition, apart from that of doctor of first contact. Consequently, the tripartite structure of the National Health Service reflected the long-entrenched divisions within the medical profession and reinforced the inferior status of the general practitioner.

2

THE DEVELOPMENT OF GENERAL PRACTICE IN THE NATIONAL HEALTH SERVICE

After 1948, general practice, with its image of structural isolation, and lack of career structure and financial incentives, contrasted strongly with the prestigious position of hospital medicine. As a result, recruitment to general practice began to decline. General practitioners became increasingly dissatisfied with a career for which they had received no training beyond their general medical education. They felt in danger of becoming mere 'sorters' in medical care, referring all complex cases to hospital doctors. They complained of patients visiting them too freely once the financial constraints to consultation were removed, of patients losing respect for them and treating them as public servants, and of the capitation system leading to poor standards of practice (Hadfield 1953; Gemmill 1958).

In response the idea of a College of General Practitioners was raised by Dr P Murphy in 1949. It was hoped that such a College would endow general practitioners with the same status as that possessed by consultants and enable them to organize themselves as a professional body. The Society of Apothecaries no longer represented the interests of these doctors and no comparable body had taken its place. The British Medical Association represented them in negotiations and in general matters, but it did not impose educational requirements. A diploma provided by a College could give general practitioners a measure of distinction as well as enhancing their professional status. The College of General Practitioners was eventually founded in 1952. By January 1963, it possessed 6200 members and associates, thirty-seven regional faculties, and three regional councils. By forming their own College, general practitioners declared themselves equal to consultants. However, they did not receive a Royal Charter, one of the essential features of professional status, until 1972 and, structurally, financially and educationally, the two branches of the profession remained unequal.

Continuing advances in medical technology further enhanced the status of hospital medicine at the expense of general practice. The low esteem of general practice was evident in Lord Moran's evidence to the Pilkington Commission in 1958. The Chairman of the Commission had said that it had been suggested that general practitioners and consultants were not junior and senior professionals, but equal. Moran (1958) replied that those doctors who entered general practice were those who had fallen off the ladder of success in hospital medicine. Curwen's (1964) study also found that only one in three doctors entered general practice of their own choice.

Three more controversial studies undertaken during this period all basically agreed that the standard of general practice needed improving (Collings 1950; Hadfield 1953; Taylor 1954). Furthermore, a study undertaken by the Association for the Study of Medical Education, for the Royal Commission on Medical Education reporting in 1968, found a relationship between students who experienced difficulty in assimilating medical knowledge and those who chose general practice as a career. In a follow-up study of this survey, it was discovered that recruits to general practice included a significantly higher proportion of students who had failed examinations (Last, Martin, and Stanley 1967). Although the 1963 Gillie Committee attempted to raise general practitioners' status by emphasizing their unique role, its arguments were not regarded as satisfactory by the profession (Report of the Sub-Committee of the Standing Medical Advisory Committee 1963). The Committee emphasized the importance of dealing with the social and psychological aspects of medicine and the significance of the general practitioner in acting as the doctor of first contact. Unfortunately, it did not specify the best way of performing the general practitioner's role, or how such doctors could best be equipped for it. It was this role and status insecurity, together with dissatisfaction over the level of remuneration, which contributed to the unrest among general practitioners in the 1960s. This eventually culminated in their threat of mass resignation from the National Health Service.

It was felt that hospital services were being improved at the expense of general practice, where list sizes were rising and the proportion of doctors was falling. Such developments were occurring at a time when the changing age structure of the population, with relatively larger proportions of elderly persons and children, was placing an increasing burden on doctors. Doctors' discontent eventually reached a climax on the issue of remuneration. The Spens Committee of 1946 suggested that the level of general practitioners' remuneration should bear the same relationship to the income of other groups as it had in 1939 (Report on General Practitioners 1946). However, the remuneration of hospital staff was considered in a separate Spens Report of 1948 and the result was an increase in the financial differential between consultants and general practitioners (Report on Consultants and Specialists 1948). Negotiations then commenced between general practitioners and the Government, which resulted in the establishment of the pool method of payment. With this, an overall sum was made available to be divided, according to certain criteria, among practitioners. In 1956, the profession sought to increase the size of the pool. It was not until these doctors threatened to withdraw from the National Health Service in 1965 that their remuneration was seriously considered by the Government. In 1963, the independent Review Body, set up after 1960 to advise the Government on doctors' remuneration, recommended an increase of 14 per cent in the level of doctors' pay. General practitioners, dissatisfied with this recommendation, pressurized the Review Body and, consequently, were awarded a further 9 per cent in 1965. The profession still considered this figure to be unsatisfactory.

The pool method of payment was increasingly regarded as a disincentive to the practice of good medicine. Doctors campaigned for its abolition and this proposal was incorporated into the British Medical Association's Charter for the Family Doctor Service of 1965. Other proposals included a five and a half day working week, six weeks' paid annual holiday, payments for out of hours' services, an independent corporation to make long-term loans to general practitioners for building and improving surgery premises, and direct reimbursement for practice expenses, ancillary help, and similar outgoings. Once again, however, concentration on practicalities obscured the basic problem of the role and status of the general practitioner in the health service.

At the height of the unrest, the Government agreed to enter into negotiations over the Charter with the profession and the threat of resignation was deferred. Long negotiations ensued which resulted in a contract embodying some, but not all, of the demands. It consisted of a basic payment available at the full rate to doctors with at least 1000 patients who provided full services for a minimum period in each week. This was available to other doctors at proportionally reduced rates. Additions were made in respect of group practice and practice in problem areas. Two levels of distinction awards were available to approximately 30 per cent of practitioners aged between 45 and 65, dependent on attendance at a required number of postgraduate training courses. Additional services provided by general practitioners, such as cervical cytology, vaccinations and immunizations, maternity and emergency work, were to be remunerated on an item for service basis. The capitation fees for ordinary week-day work were to be fixed at two rates, the rate for patients over sixty-five years of age being approximately 30 per cent higher than for other patients. Night and week-end work were additionally remunerated. An extra capitation fee for lists of over 1000 patients was made. Home visits made between midnight and seven in the morning were to be remunerated at a flat rate. Six weeks' paid holiday and a notional five-and-a-half-day working week were established on the provision that practitioners arranged for the care of their patients in their absence.

A further report from the Review Body increased the various fees and general practitioners received a further gross increase of 8 per cent. Although these doctors had not achieved all their aims, their financial position relative to consultants had been improved. Most significantly, there was now financial encouragement for the establishment of group practice from purpose-built or converted premises and for the employment of ancillary staff. Again, however, although these measures appeared to placate the profession, the wider problems of general practice still remained.

The financial and organizational changes emerging from the doctors' crisis of 1965 were the main reasons for the development of better equipped and organized general practices. The renaissance of general practice also had its origins in the increasing influence of Balint (1957) who emphasized the psycho-social causes of illness and the therapeutic potential of the doctor–patient relationship. Although his methods were popular with only a minority of doctors, they took place in an era in which the work of the general practitioner was becoming less concerned with episodes of acute illness. With the advent of antibiotics and other drugs, illness was increasingly contained before it became serious. Consequently, general practitioners were increasingly faced with treating chronic illness and social aspects of disease. This shift in emphasis was one of the reasons for the development of the concept of the team approach to care. General practice was considered too complex for the skills of any single professional. What effect have these changes had on the role and status of general practitioners?

The development of group practice

The concept of group practice operating out of health centres was recommended as long ago as 1920 in the Dawson Report (Interim Report on the Future Provision of Medical and Allied Services 1920). The British Medical Association Board of Science and Education (1974) have also pointed out the advantages of this method of organization. They stated that peer influence and informal learning within the group raise the standard of care and hence raise the status of the general practitioner. As a result doctors may find their work more satisfying. A group can afford to provide itself with better premises and equipment and with more ancillary help than is possible for a doctor working alone. They also have more opportunity to hold outside appointments as their time should be more flexible. Group practice provides a more realistic method of organization for the development of primary health care teams and has been advocated in both the Report of the Sub-Committee of the Standing Medical Advisory Committee (1963), and the Report of the Royal Commission on Medical Education (1968). Controversy still exists over one issue – the optimum number of doctors in a group.

Whatever the ideal size, however, to be more successful the model of group practice calls for a substantial reorientation in the attitudes of the medical profession. Admittedly, there has been a steady decline in single-handed practice and in group practices comprising of two or three doctors. In 1951, 80 per cent of general practitioners practised single handed. In 1971, 80 per cent of doctors practised from groups of two or more (Department of Health and Social Security, Annual Reports, 1951–1972). Such developments have been slow. Today, 40 per cent of general practitioners still practise single handed or in partnerships of only two doctors. Less than 8 per cent practise from groups of six or more, and still only 35 per cent from groups of four or more (Department of Health and Social Security, Annual Report, 1977).

Thus, although the trend is for more doctors to practise in groups, they still tend to remain in small partnerships rather than large ones. This is possibly because the concept of group practice and the primary health care team are anathema to the traditional notion of independence still respected by many doctors. However, the image of the general practitioner as totally independent, practising in isolation from other doctors and other health care workers, cannot survive if group practice and health centres are to become the standard pattern of medical practice. A study of general practice in the London

Borough of Camden indicated that some doctors *would* dislike working in teams (Sidel, Jefferys, and Masfield 1972). However, as the authors point out, general practice cannot be organized around the psychological needs of individuals who may perform best when practising alone.

The fact that more recent graduates are being educated in the value of group practice is suggested by Cartwright and Anderson's (1981) finding that doctors practising in groups tend to be younger than single-handed doctors. Perhaps this influx of recent graduates into general practice will gradually change its nature and result in its status being enhanced. The same authors found that doctors practising from groups have a more even distribution of work, have more modern, better equipped, premises, more ancillary staff, and are more likely to have access to hospital facilities as well as to hold part-time hospital appointments. Finally, it was also discovered that they are more likely to be satisfied with general practice.

Health centres

Health centres have also been advocated as a method of improving the quality and organization of general practice. The concept was clarified by the Dawson Report which pointed to the dangers of isolation in medicine (Interim Report on the Future Provision of Medical and Allied Services, 1920). The main purpose of such a centre was to provide a base for the integration of the different elements of the health service and suggestions for the implementation of health centres were incorporated into the plans for the National Health Service. However, in 1948 Bevan excused local authorities from providing such plans, possibly due to the scarcity of building resources after the war as well as the high capital costs of building the centres. A further reason may have been the hostility of general practitioners towards them.

Many doctors were suspicious of health centres, since they were afraid of being controlled by the local health authority and of losing their independence. Hadfield's (1953) survey found that health centres were popular among less than half the general practitioners questioned. However, interest in health centres has increased over the past decade or so. In 1966 the Government agreed to encourage their development by local authorities in England and Wales and by the central Government in Scotland and Northern Ireland. From 1967 to 1971, 241 new health centres were built. In 1977, there were 842 health centres in use in the United Kingdom from which 4338 doctors practised – this amounted to 20 per cent of the total number of general practitioners. In contrast, in 1965 there were twenty-eight health centres and 215 doctors practising in them (Drury 1977). Although many doctors have retained their suspicion of health centres, Irvine and Jefferys (1971) found that most health centres provide more space, equipment and staff than other types of practices. On the other hand, the initial plan to hold consultant out-patient clinics in health centres has largely failed to materialize.

The general practitioner and the hospital

Since 1965, attempts have been made to improve open access to hospital diagnostic facilities for general practitioners. Despite initial resistance from diagnostic departments, who feared an increase in inappropriate usage, studies have shown that doctors exercise discretion when making requests (Wallace *et al.* 1973). Although the number of requests is increasing, the use of diagnostic services varies widely between different general practitioners, with younger doctors and doctors in partnerships being the highest users (Loudon 1977). Cartwright and Anderson (1981) found a relationship existed between access and the possession of hospital appointments. Of the seven facilities they asked about (skeletal X-rays, barium meal X-rays, urine micro and culture, liver function tests, blood counts, electrocardiology, and physiotherapy), general practitioners with hospital appointments had access to the highest number, 5.8 on average in comparison with 5.3 of those without a hospital appointment. General practitioners' access to hospital beds is a further indicator of their relationship with, and involvement in, the hospital sector. It is also an indicator of the scientific content of their role. What changes have occurred here? General practitioner beds are located in general hospitals, maternity units, and in general practitioner hospitals. In 1955, general practitioner maternity beds accounted for 14 per cent of all maternity beds. Sixteen years later, Israel and Draper (1971) found that these beds now accounted for 22 per cent of all maternity beds. They also found that 76 per cent of general practitioner beds were completely separate from consultant hospitals, and only 6 per cent were attached to district general or specialist hospitals. They pointed out that general practitioner beds, other than maternity, represented only 3 per cent of all hospital beds (excluding psychiatric). Most of these beds are situated in cottage or smaller hospitals. The majority of these general practitioner hospitals are descendants of the 300 cottage hospitals built during the second half of the nineteenth century to serve the sick and poor in isolated areas. The Platt Report visualized their continuation as a means of maintaining continuity of care by the family doctor, in familiar surroundings close to the patient's home (Report of the Joint Working Party on the Medical Staffing Structure in the Hospital Service, 1961). However, plans were subsequently introduced to effect their closure and to concentrate services in district general hospitals (Hospital Plan, 1962; Report of the Committee on the Functions of the District General Hospital, 1969). Such plans were strongly criticized and the Hospital Plan was subsequently revised in 1966 to encourage the use of smaller hospitals.

Cartwright and Anderson (1981) found that the proportion of general practitioners with access to hospital beds in 1977 had not increased significantly since 1964. They also found that the proportion wanting beds had declined from 72 per cent in 1964 to 61 per cent in 1977. Access was higher among doctors with hospital appointments and those practising in low-density areas.

If the status of general practitioners relative to hospital doctors is to increase, then the two must understand and respect each other's roles. It does not appear that open access to diagnostic facilities or general practitioner beds has been able to significantly affect this communication process. Long and Atkins (1974) found that, in a four-week period, half the general practitioners studied had no meetings with any specialist. Cartwright and Anderson (1981) did find that the proportion of general practitioners with part-time hospital appointments had risen markedly from 23 per cent in 1964 to 40 per cent in 1977. However, the majority of practitioners still have no direct role in hospital medicine. In many cases the referral letter is the only communication between general practitioners and hospital doctors. Moreover, just as there is dissatisfaction among general practitioners concerning the style and content of consultants' letters, consultants are equally dissatisfied with the number of 'please see and advise' type of letters they receive from general practitioners (Butterfield and Wadsworth 1966). It is possible that an increasing number of domiciliary consultations may help to facilitate communications between these two branches of the profession. However, not only are few such consultations requested, but the general practitioner is not present at two-thirds of these visits (Honigsbaum 1972). Domiciliary visits are merely used to circumvent long waiting lists.

Involvement in hospital medicine may solve some of the problems of the hospital, but it does not necessarily solve problems in general practice. The lack of a direct hospital role is not necessarily of significance; what is important is the lack of meaningful contact with hospital consultants. A recent study by Whitfield (1980) found that newly appointed consultants had a very limited knowledge of the work of the general practitioner. This knowledge appears unlikely to improve. Further, while Cartwright and Anderson (1981) found that 30 per cent of general practitioners questioned felt that relationships between general practitioners and hospitals had improved over the previous ten years, 28 per cent believed they had deteriorated, and 42 per cent thought there was no change. While general practitioners do not need to play a role in hospital medicine to enhance their status, they do have to be afforded greater respect by other branches of medicine. Poor communication hampers this process.

Minor surgery in general practice

The relationship between the general practitioner and the hospital doctor may become strained, and the former accorded less respect, if hospital doctors feel that many hospital referrals are unnecessary. It has been estimated that between 33 per cent and 70 per cent of referrals to accident and emergency departments could have been treated by a general practitioner (Fry 1960; Nuffield 1960; Roy, Williams, and Bourns 1973; Holohan 1976). It has also been discovered that patients with minor ailments often refer themselves to such departments because they underestimate their own doctors' willingness to treat them, because they regard hospital medicine as better, because they are critical of their doctors, and because of poor access to general practitioners (Holohan, Newell, and Walker 1975; Gunawardena and Lee 1977; Cartwright and Anderson 1981). Undoubtedly, there is a decline in the amount of minor surgery performed in general practice. After 1948 general practitioners were finally excluded from hospital facilities for the performance of such work. Not only do most doctors' surgeries lack the equipment for performing these tasks, but general practitioners also lack the financial incentive to do it. Although health centres may be well equipped for the performance of minor surgery, general practitioners are increasingly withdrawing from this sphere (Cartwright and Anderson 1981). This is despite the recommendation of the Report of the Joint Working Party on the Medical Staffing Structure in the Hospital Service (1961) that general practitioners should relieve accident and emergency departments of this aspect of their work.

It is not only accident and emergency departments that suffer from unnecessary referrals. Approximately a quarter of referrals to consultants are referred back to general practitioners after only one consultation. Eighty-three per cent of referrals to consultant surgeons terminate with the initial interview without any pathology or X-ray investigation (Forsyth and Logan 1968). It is in the general practitioner's own interest to perform investigative and minor surgical work where possible, and not automatically refer patients to hospitals. Unnecessary referrals may lead hospital doctors to believe that general practitioners are not competent to perform many minor procedures. High rates of referral may also decrease the general practitioner's satisfaction with his or her work as contact with the patient is lost.

The primary health care team

The primary health care team generally consists of a group of people who make different contributions towards the achievement of a common goal. They do this by virtue of their diverse but related knowledge and skills. The rationale behind teams is that they facilitate the sharing of knowledge in an era in which health care is becoming so complicated that it falls outside the scope of any one branch of medicine.

The increase in the number of doctors practising from groups and the financial incentives to improve practice premises introduced in 1965 have greatly facilitated the process of different health care professionals working together at a primary care level. The 1965 measures gave doctors financial incentives to employ up to two full-time equivalent ancillary staff per principal. (A principal is a doctor providing a full range of medical services under the National Health Service.) Doctors were, and still are, reimbursed for 70 per cent of these staff members' salaries. Doctors' freedom to delegate procedures to ancillary staff was created in an amendment to their terms of service in 1966, and was later extended to cover nursing staff employed by the local health authority (now the area health authority) in a further amendment in 1972.

Why did it take so long for a team approach to primary health care to be encouraged? Part of the answer lies in the tripartite structure of the National Health Service prior to the 1974 reorganization. This structure led to administrative divisions between the various services. Hospital staff were employed by regional hospital boards; general practitioners were under contract to executive councils – they still are under contract to a separate body: family practitioner committees – and district nurses and health visitors worked in isolation, according to geographical areas, and were employed by local health authorities. After 1974, these professionals, with the exception of general practitioners, came under the umbrella of the area health authorities, which were in turn responsible to the regional health authorities. The family practitioner committees, responsible for general practitioner services, are statutory committees of the area health authorities, and are accountable to these bodies.

Prior to 1965 few doctors employed their own nurses. Because of the structural divisions described above, it took the financial incentives offered in 1965 to provide a more realistic setting for the employment and attachment of ancillary staff so that a team approach could begin to develop. However, as Reedy (1977) has pointed out, more than this was necessary for teamwork to become widespread. A reconciliation was needed between the, then, local health authorities and general practices. This reconciliation began early on when experimental attachment schemes involving health visitors were set up in Hampshire and Oxford (Swift and MacDougall 1964; Warin 1968). Attachment may be defined as staff being assigned to a general practice rather than to a geographical area. These schemes were then extended during the 1960s. In 1963 the Report of the Sub-Committee of the Standing Medical Advisory Committee suggested that domiciliary nursing staff should be attached to general practices. This suggestion was endorsed by the Royal College of Nursing and the College of General Practitioners, and, consequently, attachment schemes began to increase. The Health Services and Public Health Act of 1968 extended the sphere of action of local health authority employed nurses from patients' homes and into surgeries and clinics. This legislation also empowered local health authorities to negotiate cross-boundary visiting with neighbouring authorities. Thus, after the 1960s, doctors could not only be partly reimbursed for the salaries of privately employed ancillary staff, but could also have local health authority staff attached to their practices.

The best method of organizing a primary health care team is still unknown. Such a team is usually composed of secretarial staff, possibly an employed or attached treatment room nurse, area health authority attached staff such as a health visitor, a midwife, and a district nurse. Social workers are also occasionally attached by the local authority. The district, or community, nurse is a state registered nurse and is often assisted by a state enrolled nurse and an untrained nursing auxiliary, who often undertakes the bathing of patients. Less frequently, other staff, such as physiotherapists, psychologists, or chiropodists, may attend a health centre for certain sessions.

However, as so many doctors still practise from small units, the attachment or employment of a wide range of ancillary staff is not facilitated. Moreover, the mere presence of other health care staff in a surgery or health centre does not imply that teamwork necessarily follows. Unless the occupational groups involved understand each other's roles and the aims of the team, and unless effective channels of communication between the members exist, then a group of health care staff may not work together successfully. Gilmore, Bruce, and Hunt (1974), describing an intensive study of three health centres, in addition to their random selection of thirty-six, found that the lack of opportunity and time for adequate discussion between team members led to increased misunderstandings and frustrations. Most teams had not developed a policy with regard to communication between team members. This is largely an organizational problem. However, a lack of understanding of other members' roles is possibly the fault of education. The solution may be to integrate the training of general practitioners with other members of the team. An experimental training course for general practitioner trainees and student health visitors has been successfully conducted in Oxford. The aim of the course was to introduce these two groups in order to modify attitudes, increase knowledge of each other's work, and induce a more positive approach to teamwork in their final careers. At the end of the course over half the participants stated that they had a better grasp of the other's role (Hasler and Klinger 1976).

One issue which often leads to conflict within teams is the question of who should head the team. The sharing of skills may be an essential feature of teamwork, but does this sharing imply equality between the personnel concerned or should one professional be singled out to lead the team? Dingwall (1976) has shown that the issue of leadership is viewed in different ways by different types of personnel. For example, while health visitors define the team in a non-hierarchical sense, general practitioners see it as a group of auxiliary workers to be organized and directed by the doctor. In practice, teamwork in primary care, in so far as it exists, is influenced by the traditional model of medical dominance, as well as that of traditional female sub-servience to males – most doctors are men and members of most occupations ancillary to medicine are traditionally female. It is understandably difficult for general practitioners to break away from a pattern of dominance. They have been trained in a hospital setting where the nurse's subordination to the doctor is much in evidence. Moreover, on the issue of leadership in primary care doctors have several advantages over other health care staff. As McIntosh and Dingwall (1978) have pointed out, the doctor is the person who establishes the practice and thus wishes to control personal resources. Further, the doctor is the staff member who is finally responsible for the well-being of the patient.

Although other staff are legally responsible for their own actions, general practitioners may still feel that their overall responsibility entitles them to hold the role of team leader. This view may be reinforced by the fact that only doctors are equipped to perform the essential function of general practice as it is presently organized: diagnosis and treatment. On the other hand, it could be argued that the complex nature of the team's activities calls for many acts of leadership which no one person can provide. Perhaps the issue of who should lead the primary health care team, if anyone, should be left for individual teams to decide. Some teams may prefer a clearly defined leader and a hierarchical ordering of authority, whilst others may opt for a more egalitarian approach. However, the issue is often not so much that of who should lead the team, but how to persuade doctors to operate within a team framework at all. To what extent do general practitioners work with other health care staff? The team approach to primary care does not appear to have progressed very far, since the only health workers to be attached to general practices on a wide scale are district nurses and health visitors. Where only two types of personnel, apart from administrative staff, work alongside the doctor one must question whether the use of the term team is a justifiable description of their functioning, especially in view of the fact that working together physically does not ensure a team approach to care.

Secretaries and receptionists

Administrative staff, such as secretaries, receptionists and practice managers are usually employed by the general practitioner, except in the case of health centres where they may be attached by the area health authority. Doctors have responded dramatically to the financial incentives offered them in the mid-1960s to employ ancillary staff. Although they rarely have practice managers, Cartwright and Anderson (1981) found that all except four doctors, 1 per cent, in their sample said they had a secretary or receptionist, in comparison with a quarter who did not have one in Cartwright's (1967) earlier survey. These authors found that the average number of secretaries in a practice was four, the number increasing with the number of doctors in the group. However, it has been argued (Drury and Kuenssberg 1970) that many doctors do not always take optimum advantage of the skills of these personnel.

Health visitors

During the nineteenth century, when infectious diseases were a major health problem, the health visitor's role concentrated mainly on the teaching of hygiene. By the early twentieth century, the high infant mortality rate became a source of medical concern and the role of the health visitor, reflecting this difference in emphasis, centred on ensuring maternal and infant welfare. With rising standards of living and improvements in standards of health in the post-war period, health visiting began to move towards the psycho-social needs of children and families. Today, health visitors are registered nurses who have received a twelve-month training qualifying them to give health education, advice and counselling to maternity patients, women with small children and, to a lesser extent, the elderly. It has been found, however, that health visitors lack a sense of professional identity because they feel they have too many duties to give enough time to any one task in particular (Hunt 1972).

As early as 1956, the Report of the Working Party on the Field of Work, Training and Recruitment of Health Visitors recommended that health visitors should work more closely with general practitioners in order to help eliminate the demarcation line between curative and preventive medicine. The rate of attachment of health visitors to general practices is slightly higher than that of district nurses and health visitors actually preceded nurses in attachment schemes. In contrast to the mid-1960s when few health visitors were attached to general medical practices, the proportion is now 79 per cent (Reedy 1977).

The role of the health visitor has long been misunderstood by doctors, despite their high rates of attachment. Jefferys (1965) found that half the general practitioners in her survey of Buckinghamshire made critical comments about health visitors. These comments reflected much ignorance about the precise nature of the health visitor's function. This confusion is reinforced by treatment room nurses taking over preventive work such as immunizations and 'well baby clinics', tasks traditionally performed by health visitors. There is also a certain amount of role overlap between health visitors and social workers which leads to further misunderstandings and ambiguities.

Midwives

Midwifery is an ancient art. Midwives were licensed as early as the sixteenth century, soon after the 1512 Act aiming at the regulation of medicine and surgery, although it was not until 1902 that the Midwives' Act, regulating the profession, became law.

The attachment of midwives to general practice has been affected by the declining number of home as opposed to hospital births, the consequent changing role of the general practitioner in relation to obstetrics, and the declining national birth rate. The hospital confinement rate has been increasing since the late 1950s and was reinforced by the Peel Report (Report of the Sub-Committee of the Standing Maternity and Midwifery Advisory Committee 1970). This recommended that most women should have their babies in hospital. Over 90 per cent of births now take place in hospital (Department of Health and Social Security 1980b). The report foresaw midwives being increasingly attached to hospitals, and it appears that this has been happening. From 1971 to 1973 the number of domiciliary midwives in England fell by almost 900 to a total of 4855, a reduction of approximately 6 per cent a year. There was a corresponding reduction in the ratio of midwives to general practitioners (Department of Health and Social Security 1974). As a result of these changes, the domiciliary midwife, whose function is to provide care throughout pregnancy, labour, and the lying-in period, is also experiencing role ambiguity.

Social workers

The Report of the Committee on Local Health Authority and Allied Personal Social Services (1968), as well as recommending the integration of the previously fragmented branches of the social services, pointed out that doctors had been slow in taking advantage of the relatively new profession of social work. It stated that social workers had a valuable contribution to make in dealing with psychological and social factors in the management of illness and in its prevention. The report did not recommend the attachment of social workers to general practice, as it did not feel that general practitioners were ready for such a development. However, in 1974, the British Medical Association Report on Primary Health Care Teams stated that the organization of general practice should include social workers. Goldberg and Neill (1972) have pointed to a number of studies which indicate that doctors have infrequent, if any, contact with such personnel. Ratoff (1973) discovered that less than half of the social services departments he studied in 1972 had social workers who had any involvement with general practitioners while Cartwright and

Anderson (1981) found that 23 per cent of their sample of general practitioners said they had an attached social worker. They feel that this figure is an exaggeration as doctors did not distinguish between the term attachment and liaison. However, just over half of the doctors in their study who said they did not have an attached social worker also said that they would like one. However, social workers still seem to be less popular among doctors than nurses: a situation that is not helped by the fact that only 37 per cent of social workers hold a recognized qualification in social work (Reedy 1977). Furthermore, there is much role confusion between social workers and health visitors. Perhaps the main. distinctions between these two types of health personnel are the lack of a medical background among social workers, which may partly explain the reluctance of many doctors to work with them, and the intensive casework approach which is typical of their method. Thus, social worker attachments to general practice still seem to be at an experimental stage, at least in comparison with other attachment schemes. Given the acute staffing problems in many social service departments, social workers may be as unready as many general practitioners to develop such schemes fully.

Nursing staff

The situation regarding nursing staff is more complicated because of their dual roles and employers. A distinction exists between a nurse who is privately employed and a nurse who is employed by the area health authority and attached to a general practice. While the former type of nurse has traditionally worked mainly in the surgery, the attached nurse has worked mainly in the patient's home. Reedy (1977) has pointed out that this distinction is now becoming slightly blurred, as attached nurses transfer more of their work into the surgery. This practice saves their visiting time, in the case of patients who are mobile, and they are also finding themselves performing more delegated medical procedures. Moreover, in the case of health centres, area health authorities attach nurses specifically to work in treatment rooms. The distinction between these two types of nurse has its origins in the occasional private employment of nurses by doctors before 1948. In contrast, district nurses have their origins in community nursing services which were increasingly provided by voluntary associations before 1948 in response to the public health movement. The introduction of the National Health Service reinforced this distinction, as the 1946 Act confined the then local health authority employed nurses to working in patients' homes, a constraint which has only recently been removed. Today, district nurses, who are state registered nurses in the case of sisters, or state enrolled nurses, have usually received a short course of in-service training to equip them for working in patients' homes. As a result of the recommendations of the Report of the Committee on Nursing (1972), this training will become compulsory for district nurses from 1981.

Nursing attachments to general practice appear popular among doctors. Although there has been a steady increase in the numbers of district nurses and although approximately 77 per cent of them are attached to general practice, only 68 per cent of practices in England have at least one attached nurse (Reedy, Philips, and Newell 1976; Department of Health and Social Security 1980b). Furthermore, while Reedy, Philips, and Newell (1976) found that 89 per cent of practices with four or five principals had attached nurses, this was true of only 51 per cent of all single-handed practices. There are also significant regional variations in attachment rates. Even though attachment schemes are relatively widespread, apart from among single-handed practitioners, the private employment of nurses by doctors is also continuing to increase. These authors have shown that general practitioners in England were employing just over 3100 nurses in 1974. Again, the employment of nurses was found to increase with the number of doctors in the practice. However, the number of such nurses is small in comparison with the number of general practitioners in England, which is over 24 000 (Department of Health and Social Security, Annual Report 1977). From the doctors' point of view, privately employed nurses have the advantage of lack of external constraints on their activities, unlike attached nurses, and they also complement the doctor's conception of independence. Moreover, although their activities overlap to some extent, it has been found that attached nurses still perform more caring functions (bathing, feeding, cleansing of patients) than technical activities (ear syringing, venepuncture), in contrast to the privately employed nurse (Reedy *et al.* 1980b).

Nursing and health authorities themselves disapprove of the concept of the nurse privately employed by the general practitioner. Not only is such a nurse responsible to a member of another profession, but the dual employment of nurses may sometimes create legal problems in the event of a mishap. The privately employed nurse may not only receive no encouragement to undertake adequate insurance protection, but such nurses may also believe themselves absolved from responsibility for their actions. While nursing bodies would probably like to see all nurses employed by the health authorities for these reasons, Marsh and Kaim Caudle (1976) have even suggested that the state registered nurse employed as a district nurse could delegate nursing functions to a state enrolled nurse and, instead, adopt a role which is supervisory in addition to undertaking tasks currently performed by the doctor. Such a suggestion dispenses with the privately employed nurse, who is superseded by the state registered community nurse. Whether community nurses would want such a dramatic change in their role is another matter, apart from the fact that it would place them under greater medical subordination.

However, although controversy over role divisions may be inevitable, doctors' skills could undoubtedly be better utilized if they had the opportunity to work with other occupational groups. In addition, attachment schemes should result in more contact between different types of health workers and assist them in developing broader perspectives of health care. Although the attachment of health visitors to general practice may be developing its preventive aspects, and the employment and attachment of nurses may be enabling doctors to discard the non-medical aspects of their role, it is difficult to foresee how attachment schemes and employment trends can have much impact on the doctors' role and status until a greater variety of ancillary staff work from their premises. Roles also need to be clarified in order that maximum use may be made of each person's skills. Moreover, as we have previously noted, physical proximity does not imply a team approach to care. Studies of general practice are needed in order to assess to what extent various types of personnel actually collaborate with each other, rather than simply operating from the same practice premises.

3

THE ROLE AND STATUS OF THE
GENERAL PRACTITIONER TODAY

In contrast to the situation in the 1960s, there has been a large increase in the number of new entrants to general practice. It is now apparently the most popular career choice among medical students (Parkhouse 1979). Is this due to an increase in status because of the organizational improvements in general practice? Studies in the United States have shown no relationship between the perceived status of a specialty and specialty choice (Matteson and Smith 1977). Moreover, over half the general practitioners in Cartwright and Anderson's (1981) survey thought that the relative prestige of general practice in the medical profession had not changed over the last ten years. Only one third felt it had risen. In addition, twice as many of the patients in their study thought that general practitioners' prestige had gone down in the last ten years as thought it had gone up. A comparison of Cartwright's (1967) findings in 1964 with those of this later study showed that general practitioners' assessments of the extent to which they enjoy their work had hardly changed. In fact, a lower proportion of those in the later study said that they enjoyed it at all. It appears that the increased popularity of general practice among medical students may simply be due to its improved levels of remuneration.

The need for a body of knowledge in general practice

The problem of general practice still seems to be its lack of role definition based on an independent body of knowledge – a prerequisite of full professional status. The problem is partly attributable to a paucity of research in general practice and lack of adequate postgraduate training facilities. The many official and government reports on general practice have failed in their attempts to provide this definition. In 1950 a British Medical Association Committee emphasized the importance of treating the whole person. In 1954 the Report of the Committee of the Central Health Services Council laid down several functions of the general practitioner, including continuing responsibility for patients' health; diagnosis, treatment and management of conditions treatable in the home; referral to hospital when necessary; preventive medicine, health education and supervision of convalescence; emergency treatment; and administrative and legal functions. In 1963 the Report of the Subcommittee of the Standing Medical Advisory Committee affirmed the significant role of the general practitioner, particularly in the area of treating behavioural problems and the co-ordination of patient care. Apart from recommending improvements in practice organization, this report simply suggested that, in order to enhance its status, general practice should become a specialty in its own right, if only as that branch of medicine which did not specialize. The Report of the Royal Commission on Medical Education in 1968 emphasized the technical, rather than the pastoral, role of the general practitioner and again suggested that it should aim for specialty status. Although these basic roles have continually been emphasized, the crucial issue regarding professional status – the creation of an independent body of knowledge – has been ignored. The various reports have merely defined such doctors as the family doctor, the doctor of first contact, and as the specialist generalist. Nor does the definition of the general practitioner's work recently adopted by the Royal College of General Practitioners go far beyond these basic descriptions (Joint Committee on Postgraduate Training for General Practice 1976).

Is it in the interests of health care provision and patients' needs for general practitioners to aim for such a body of knowledge? If these doctors lack status and direction without this knowledge, and hence have no secure role, then morale may be low and, consequently, so may be standards of practice. This question, however, demands an analysis of the alternative roles and knowledge bases open to general practitioners. How can the doctor's time be used best? What needs for medical care exist? How can medical input and output be better equated?

Needs may be defined in terms of the existence of illness or disabilities, and demands in terms of individuals considering that they have needs and wish to receive care. Needs are not necessarily expressed as demands and demands are not necessarily followed by utilization. On the other hand, demand and utilization may exist

without needs. These definitions are to some extent oversimplifi-
cations. Concepts of need are imbued with value judgments. An
individual may recognize a need which may or may not coincide with
a professional's definition. Nor do medical definitions of need necessarily coincide. The patient's definition of need may be influenced by
various social and psychological factors. On the professional's part,
resource limitations may influence decisions and interpretations.
Demand is potentially unlimited. For every person who seeks medical
help, there are far more who treat themselves, or who tolerate their
symptoms (Wadsworth, Butterfield, and Blaney 1971). Although
self-reliance is to be encouraged, in an era of rising expectations there
will always be many competing demands for limited health care
resources. Thus the question of priorities is raised. With increasing
health care costs, not only must the most efficient methods of
organizing primary medical care be taken into account, but the
doctor's role must also be considered in terms of health needs. The
scope for the expansion of the doctor's technical role in the surgery
has been considered. There is a need, for example, for doctors to
undertake more minor surgical procedures in general practice and to
perform more thorough examinations of patients before referring
them to hospital departments. Such practices could enable out-
patient departments to concentrate their costly resources on more
appropriate, complex cases.

Are there any further areas of need in which general practitioners
could expand their role and which could also contribute to the
formulation of a more exclusive body of knowledge? Greater concentration on technical aspects of medicine does not necessarily satisfy
these criteria, as it is often largely an extension of hospital medicine.
One model of health care which is sometimes suggested as an area of
need on which general practitioners might concentrate are the socio-
psychological aspects of medicine. Recently, for example, the Report
of the Royal Commission on the National Health Service (1979)
recommended more training in psychological aspects of medicine for
general practitioners. However, Stimson (1977) has pointed to the
many ambiguities inherent in such terms. For example, he states that
the social element in general practice could refer to the doctor–
patient relationship; awareness of social factors in disease and illness
behaviour; awareness of social welfare problems, and the doctor's role
in treating emotional problems in the socio-psychotherapeutic role.
Medical discussions of socio-psychological aspects of medicine tend
to concentrate on the latter definition. However, many general
practitioners lack interest in this aspect of medicine. Cartwright and

Anderson (1981) found that the proportion of doctors who feel that it is appropriate for people to seek help from their general practitioners for problems in their family lives fell from 87 per cent in Cartwright's (1967) earlier study to 67 per cent in 1977. Doctors in 1977 were also less likely to feel that it was reasonable for patients to consult them over personal problems. Moreover, it was the older, rather than the younger, doctors who felt that such consultations were appropriate.

Although mental health is as important as physical health, it could be argued that general practitioners may not be interested in developing their therapeutic potential in this area unless they can perceive specific advantages for themselves in so doing. One such advantage could be the development of their own body of knowledge in this area. No progress, however, will be made without research and one main problem in general practice is poor clinical research. In the field of counselling in general practice, Balint (1957) has illustrated that there is no clear statement of methodology which can be taught with confidence. Of course, one problem with developing the doctor's role in this field is that it will overlap with that of the psychiatrist, psychologist, social worker, and other trained professionals. Thus, the body of knowledge it would be based upon would not be unique, and would not satisfy the criteria of professionalism. On the other hand, theories, such as psychoanalytic theories, can be reinterpreted to distinguish them from those utilized by other professionals. For example, the counselling techniques utilized by the social workers are not designed to explore the unconscious self, as are those of the psychoanalyst. The social worker's counselling skills are more basic, designed to explore emotional problems which reveal themselves in the conscious self. If general practitioners could develop their own counselling techniques and theory then they would not be infringing directly upon the methods favoured by others, at least less so than they would by concentration on technical aspects of medicine, such as minor surgery.

The Balints (M. and E. Balint 1961) themselves attached great significance to the difference between the setting of general practice and the hospital or clinic setting of psychiatrists and psychoanalysts. Specialist settings cannot achieve the continuity of care possible in a general practice setting. The consultant's contact with the patient is essentially transient and little knowledge may be gained about the patient's background and social support system. Thus, the previously mentioned superficial definitions of the general practitioner's role – such as the personal, family doctor, and the provider of continuous care – may be of crucial importance in distinguishing between the role of the general practitioner and the role of the hospital doctor – but only once the former's theoretical role has been clearly defined. Such basic definitions are still inadequate on their own.

The doctor–patient relationship is also of significance in discussions on socio-psychological aspects of medicine involving counselling. The development of a successful counselling technique necessitates a good doctor–patient relationship since patients need encouragement to talk freely. However, it is often argued that general practitioners lack the time to talk to their patients (Horder 1977; Gray 1980). The average patient consulting time in general practice is five to six minutes (Royal College of General Practitioners 1973). This is insufficient to get to know patients well and to offer any form of counselling service. Doctors often complain that they have insufficient time to treat patients who are ill, because they see so many trivial conditions. Cartwright (1967) found that the presentation of such conditions was the most frequent cause of dissatisfaction among general practitioners. Cartwright and Anderson (1981), moreover, found that the proportion of consultations doctors define as trivial, unnecessary, or inappropriate was estimated to be, on average, one-third of all consultations in the 1977 study, the same proportion as in the 1964 study. However, Cartwright (1967) felt, with some supporting evidence, that doctors tend to exaggerate the amount of trivia seen. Because general practitioners have been trained in a hospital setting, their concept of the interesting case has been defined by the hospital specialist. When they enter general practice and are confronted with problems they are not equipped to treat, their reaction may understandably be one of frustration. This belief among doctors that trivial illness is somehow not 'real' medicine cannot be conducive to the creation of a good doctor–patient relationship in general practice. Such a relationship is not easy to achieve.

Mechanic (1968) has argued that its success is often attributable to the extent that doctor and patient share common frames of reference. Difficulties are inevitable when approximately 80 per cent of doctors come from social classes one and two, in contrast to the majority of the population. Many other barriers to effective communication exist. Stimson and Webb (1975) have examined territorial, social, cultural and educational barriers, and the constraint of time on the doctor–patient relationship. Such barriers lead to an imbalance of power which leaves the patient in a weakened bargaining position. It is a sad reflection on the state of general practice and on the quality of the doctor–patient relationship that doctors appear to be more satisfied with consultations which take less than five minutes, in which the patient asks no more than one question, and in which fewer problems are discussed (Cartwright and O'Brien 1976). Other studies have indicated that medical students prefer organically ill patients, and that general practitioners are neither willing nor equipped to treat social and emotional aspects of illness (Stroller and Geertsma 1958; Reynolds and Bice 1971; Clyne 1974). However, Stimson (1976) found that although general practitioners do not like this aspect of their work, they do not necessarily wish to relinquish it.

If doctors do not enjoy non-clinical aspects of medicine, is the development of socio-psychological medicine merely a suggestion forwarded by academics for the purpose of enhancing doctors' status? Or is it a legitimate area of work for general practitioners? The need for the development of a counselling role in general practice is supported by the work of Shepherd and his colleagues (1966), who found a high consulting rate for psychological problems in general practice. Also, taking depression alone, Fry (1974) has estimated that there are 400 depressed persons in the average practice population of 2500. Of these, 100 will consult their general practitioners annually, two to three suicide attempts will occur annually, and one suicide will occur every four years. Cartwright and Anderson (1981) found that 30 per cent of patients are likely to regard general practitioners as appropriate for dealing with family and relationship problems, 28 per cent would turn to their general practitioners with a personal problem, and 69 per cent would consult them over a constant feeling of depression. As psychotropic drugs form the largest group of prescribed medicines, the development of counselling techniques by doctors as a possible alternative form of therapy could be beneficial for patients.

Psychotherapeutic techniques are not always seen as advantageous. It is maintained that one of the goals of psychotherapy is to readjust the patient's external behaviour with significant people in his or her environment (Balint 1957). This goal appears incompatible with attempts to influence the social and political environment which may be a cause of the complaint. Such approaches place the blame for ill health on the individual rather than on social, political, and economic conditions. Stimson (1977) has pointed out that it is difficult for doctors to act politically when their basic work object is the individual, and their methods are inherent in the one-to-one consultation. On the other hand, there is no reason why doctors could not lend support to local campaigns for improved housing, working conditions, and a better environment while still offering therapeutic counselling for those who need it. Therapy does not have to aim at behaviour change and personal blame. The opportunity to simply talk about problems to a professional figure may be therapeutic in itself.

Since therapeutic listening may help people develop a degree of self-awareness, this is not necessarily concomitant with acceptance of a particular social situation.

One argument against the adoption of a counselling role by general practitioners is that it increases the medicalization of life. Illich (1975) has pointed to our increasing dependency on medicine. Should an individualized approach based on self-help be emphasized instead of counselling techniques? Can the two approaches be adopted simultaneously without conflict? People should be encouraged to participate in their own health care and solve their own problems where this is possible. But a point may be reached where they will want to seek professional advice and this should not be withheld. Self-help alone is not always enough. On the other hand, the public should also not be misled into believing that professional counselling techniques have any scientifically proven value.

Is the general practitioner the best person to provide counselling, or should such methods be left to other types of professionals, or even informed lay persons? Balint (1957) did not consider the provision of counselling by a team approach or even by self-help groups. To some extent, members of self-help groups can offer each other sympathetic listening and advice. However, there may come a point when the help of someone who is trained in counselling techniques and experienced in dealing with social and emotional problems may be needed. The issue of which type of professional could best provide this care is unresolved. The best way to adopt a team approach to this branch of medicine has yet to be determined, although the role conflicts between psychiatrists, psychologists, and social workers in a hospital setting have been documented by Goldie (1977). It could be argued that the general practitioner should develop a counselling role, as there should be no dichotomy between the treatment of patients' physical conditions and their emotional and social states. The present counselling role of social workers is certainly inadequate in terms of providing this form of therapy as it has a more practical orientation. This suggests that there is scope for the development of such a role by the general practitioner.

It has been suggested by the Royal College of General Practitioners (1972) that the general practitioner should also be concerned with social factors influencing health and disease in a wider sense. For example, they could concentrate on preventive medical techniques.

The National Health Service has done little to develop preventive medicine since traditional medicine in our society is crisis medicine. It deals with disease which has already occurred and prevention is generally limited to techniques such as vaccination. Our curative medical system is based on an engineering approach to disease. This assumes that the body is a machine and that malfunctions of its separate parts can be corrected by discrete surgical, chemical, or other means. It ignores the social context of disease as well as preventive measures. It intervenes after the event, rather than before, treating the illness rather than the environmental context affecting the illness. Much of the ill health we experience can be eliminated only by changing our system of social organization and by avoiding situations which lead to stress and encourage harmful activities. There has recently been a greater interest in prevention and non-medical forms of help and this has led to a proliferation of self-help groups and literature on prevention and self-care.

The Department of Health and Social Security has also renewed its interest in this field, mainly owing to the high costs of providing health care and increasing demands for such care. However, the Department of Health and Social Security's (1976a) publication 'Prevention and Health: Everybody's Business' puts the onus for prevention on the individual and ignores the vast sums of money spent by advertisers on encouraging disease-forming habits. But what role can the general practitioner play here? Doctors are restricted mainly to giving personal advice; as a result, problems are individualized. Once again there is no reason why doctors could not become involved in local community action groups, adding strength to campaigns against environmental pollution, and poor living standards and working conditions. Doctors' time may be more effectively spent on encouraging healthy lifestyles in their local communities, than on working as an assistant in a hospital one day a week.

Even trends in personal health education in general practice are not encouraging. For most doctors, health education in practical terms simply means putting up posters in their waiting rooms (Pike 1969). A survey made by Dunnell and Cartwright (1972) suggested that only a minority of doctors thought their role specifically included health education. The fact that personalized health education does have an important place in general practice has been demonstrated by a study of five practices in which doctors gave patients advice to stop smoking. The results suggested that any general practitioner who adopts this approach could expect approximately twenty-five long-term annual successes. Thus, if all general practitioners in the

United Kingdom participated then half a million people a year would stop smoking, despite pressure from advertisers (Russell *et al.* 1979).

A further role the general practitioner may play in prevention is screening. Screening is the detection of previously unrecognized disorders by routine examination of large groups of people. Although community surveys of morbidity have detected vast amounts of untreated disease, it is questionable how much of this needs to be detected and treated. Multiphasic screening is generally regarded as wasteful in terms of time and money, although strong cases have been made in favour of the partial screening of disorders such as hypertension. Although the evidence is as yet unresolved, screening through home visiting may be an effective way of detecting hypertension (Trafford *et al.* 1979). However, a pronounced trend towards any type of regular screening programme will require a change of attitude on the part of both patient and doctor. A change in emphasis in medical education will be necessary if the recommendations of the Royal Commission on the National Health Service (1979) on the expansion of proven screening programmes are to be effected. Better use of ancillary staff and wider delegation may also be necessary if doctors are to have time to expand their roles in such directions. Much can be taken on by non-physicians. For example, in the United States, trained physicians' assistants, with the aid of protocols, even manage routine clinics for diabetes and hypertension screening themselves, simply referring positive diagnoses to the doctor. Komaroff and his colleagues (1974) found they could manage almost two-thirds of patient visits without any assistance.

More emphasis on the social and preventive aspects of the general practitioner's role may lead to a better ratio between medical input and output. Despite vast increases in the number of National Health Service staff and expenditure, and despite the development of thousands of new drugs, medical care is still not able to offer a cure for today's major medical problems. We are no longer faced with incurable infections; instead we are faced with the diseases of modern society which may be preventable but are not yet curable. Among these are heart disorders, bronchitis, the cancers, and mental disorders. What is needed, in particular, is for general practitioners to work towards a reduction of the mystique of medicine and encourage people to take an interest in the functioning and care of their own bodies, as well as the effects on them of the society in which we live.

Thus, areas of medicine do exist in which the general practitioner, and other members of the team, could play a valuable role and which could be made unique to primary care. The existing definitions of the general practitioner's role are not only superficial, but are also being increasingly usurped. For example, that of the doctor of first contact is often dispensed with by patients referring themselves to various out-patient departments such as accident and emergency and venereology. Even the role of the general practitioner as the provider of continuous care is being threatened because of increasing population mobility. In such circumstances, the 'family' doctor cannot always fully understand patients' backgrounds, nor appreciate the way in which individual circumstances may affect illness. The concept of personal doctoring has lost much of its meaning with the increasing use of deputizing services and the sharing of patients between partners in group practices. Appointment systems and ancillary staff are further factors distancing doctor and patient, in addition to the reduction in home visiting. General practitioners can no longer depend on such definitions to provide them with their role.

The current status of the general practitioner

General practitioners' status is currently as uncertain as their role. Undoubtedly, despite Cartwright and Anderson's (1981) pessimistic findings on this issue, there have been improvements in their position, perhaps the most recent example of which is the Medical Act of 1978, which permits the Royal College of General Practitioners to have a nominated member on the General Medical Council as of right. In addition, the Vocational Training Act (1977) makes vocational training for general practitioners compulsory from 1981. Future practitioners will have undergone a minimum of four years' postgraduate experience in supervised training posts. However, training in general practice is still shorter than in other branches of medicine. While it is the aim of the Royal College of General Practitioners to set a standard of competence through its membership examination, and examination is now virtually the sole means of membership to the College, only one-third of all general practitioners are Fellows, members, or associates of the College (Horder 1977). Thus the degree of professional control is still low in comparison with other specialties. General practitioners became part of a unified medical profession at the expense of remaining at the bottom of the medical hierarchy. The Royal Colleges of the various specialties safeguard standards of practice within their disciplines, but general practice has been slow in doing likewise. The only premises which have been inspected, for example, are those of the minority of practitioners who have applied to become trainers (Joint Committee on Postgraduate Training for General Practice 1976).

The uncertain position of the general practitioner is further threatened by the increasingly uncertain position of medicine as a whole. The effectiveness of modern medicine is often being questioned. Medicine has provided no cure for the diseases of industrial society; medical procedures such as tonsillectomy, inguinal hernia repair, hysterectomy, bilateral oophorectomy, and cholecystectomy are of questionable value (Radical Statistics Health Group 1977). Moreover, medicine's claim to professional status on the grounds of uniformity of opinion and solidarity are less defensible as specialties proliferate and result in differing bodies of medical opinion.

The autonomy of the medical profession is also being questioned by the medical division of labour. Medicine has always indirectly controlled other health practitioners by controlling their knowledge base. However, the situation has been gradually changing. Although the medical profession has a majority on the Central Council for the Professions Supplementary to Medicine, medical control of paramedical education is being challenged by the inclusion of non-medical subjects into the latter's degree and diploma courses, and by the intrusion of graduates in non-medical subjects into the health service. Furthermore, the political power of the trade unions has strengthened the position of other health workers in relation to the medical profession. A relatively recent example is the series of ancillaries' disputes whereby the latter became involved in decision-making in previously medical matters – for example, on the issue of what constitutes a medical emergency. Even junior hospital doctors have departed from the traditional concept of professionalism by attempting to enter into direct negotiation over wages on employer–employee lines. They have negotiated a contract which specifies the number of hours to be worked and which incorporates overtime payments. This adoption of trade union tactics may lead to a reduction in medical mystique by leading the public to view doctors as ordinary human beings. As such mystique diminishes, and as public awareness of the limitations of medicine increases, then Friedson's third condition for autonomy – public credence of the medical profession – also diminishes (Freidson 1970).

The strength of the medical profession has also been weakened by the 1974 reorganization of the National Health Service which led to an increase in administrative rather than medical control at all levels. Nurses, too, have more control. The 1974 Act also created consumer bodies, community health councils, to advise dissatisfied consumers of health care and to suggest improvements in the health service. The development of consumer representation is a threat to doctors' autonomy, despite these councils' lack of executive power and responsibility. Thus, although the medical profession is still well represented in the reorganized National Health Service, this representation has been reduced relative to other groups.

How can the status of the general practitioner be enhanced, in this climate, in a manner compatible with health service needs? The solution, it seems, still lies in clearly defining the unique contribution of the general practitioner to our health care system. This, in turn, depends on a strong tradition of clinical research and sound clinical training in this field, both of which are lacking at present. Shortage of time within general practice is often blamed for the lack of experimentation and research. One method of organization which might give doctors more time and which might lead to a more efficient utilization of skills is delegation. However, in view of the role and status threats experienced by general practitioners, they may not react favourably to any attempts to transfer medical functions to non-medical personnel. But to what extent is there a need for further delegation in general practice?

4

THE NEED FOR DELEGATION IN
GENERAL PRACTICE

It might be argued that the necessity for further delegation is partly dependent on the future supply of doctors. A future under-supply of doctors may necessitate reviewing present methods of organization. A future over-supply may obviate any need for delegation to other health workers, as this would reduce doctors' employment prospects at a time when these would be most needed. An assessment of manpower needs and supply requires an analysis of current workload trends. First, however, what is the medical manpower situation in general practice and in Britain as a whole?

Manpower trends in general practice

In contrast to the situation in the 1960s, the number of general practitioner principals has been increasing by approximately 250 a year since 1972. In 1963 there were 20 335 doctors in general practice. Today there are over 24 000.

During the 1960s general practice was an unpopular career choice according to a survey conducted by Last and Stanley (1968). Although certain studies (Parkhouse and McLaughlin 1976; Parkhouse and Howard 1978) have shown an increase in the popularity of general practice among medical students, variations between medical schools suggest that individual teachers may influence career choice. We still do not know whether larger numbers of doctors are entering general practice because it is more satisfying as a career or because the level of remuneration is higher than in junior hospital posts. It should be noted that the recent increase in the number of new recruits to general practice has been mainly due to the increase in the number of overseas doctors entering this branch of medicine. At present, approximately 15 per cent of all general practitioner principals were born overseas. With the introduction of more stringent entrance tests for immigrant doctors, the number of such entrants is declining. Will a future increase in the number of medical students compensate for fewer immigrants entering general practice, especially in inner city areas? The answer seems to be – only if doctors choose to enter general practice rather than other branches of medicine and in preference to emigrating. Of course, even more doctors may enter general practice in the future if the threatened over-supply of doctors becomes a reality. How optimistic is the future of general practice in terms of available manpower?

Conditions in general practice, and in remuneration levels, have improved considerably since 1965. Have they improved sufficiently to compete with more lucrative appointments abroad? This question cannot be given a straightforward answer, since it seems that the number of appointments abroad open to British doctors is decreasing as other countries produce more of their own doctors (Maynard and Walker 1978). However, earlier data indicated that only one-quarter of the doctors who emigrated during the 1960s were general practitioners (Abel Smith and Gales 1964). On the other hand, their data did indicate that those doctors who emigrated saw general practice as a low-status occupation in Britain at that time. Moreover, those who had not emigrated but had chosen other specialties had clearly rejected general practice as a career. Current emigration figures also suggest that many doctors still reject general practice as a career in this country. As a quarter of general practitioners in Britain are over the age of fifty-five and 6 per cent are over sixty-five, the issue becomes one of whether sufficient doctors will enter general practice in the future to replace those who retire.

The problem is particularly serious in large urban areas, such as Inner London, which have higher proportions of older doctors. Nor does the threatened situation of a general over-supply of doctors reduce the scale of the problem. Unemployed doctors are not necessarily persuaded to enter unattractive practices. Moreover, despite an increase in the number of entrants to general practice, a regional maldistribution of general practitioners still exists. An alleged shortage of doctors in many parts of Britain was one of the main problems confronting the newly created National Health Service in 1948. One of its aims was to achieve a more equitable distribution of medical care resources. Prohibitions on the buying and selling of practices were introduced, financial incentives were given to those willing to practise in under-doctored areas, and corresponding restraints were imposed in over-doctored areas. These measures had some effect in redistributing general practitioners more evenly throughout the regions. However, the proportion of National Health Service patients who resided in areas designated as under-doctored by the Medical Practices Committee still rose from 17 per cent in 1961 to 37 per cent in 1968. Basic practice allowances in officially designated under-doctored areas were increased in the mid-1960s. This had the effect of reducing list sizes to some extent; but although the gap between the regions was narrowed, the lowest list sizes are still in South-West England, where needs are probably lowest, and highest list sizes are still to be found in the Midlands and the industrial North, where needs are probably greatest. Public policy in this area since 1946 has been discussed more fully by Butler, Bevan, and Taylor (1973).

Medical manpower planning

Medical manpower in general practice cannot be considered in isolation from medical manpower planning as a whole. What are the determinants of this planning in Britain? Over the previous four decades British medical manpower policies have been affected by the recommendations of various committees. In 1944, when medical schools were admitting approximately 1850 undergraduates a year, the Report of the Interdepartmental Committee on Medical Schools (the Goodenough Report) stated that we had too few doctors. It suggested an intake target of 2500. By the mid-1950s, the medical profession was becoming alarmed at the prospect of a surplus of doctors and, in 1957, the Report of the Committee to Consider the Future Numbers of Medical Practitioners (Willink Report) advised a reduction in medical school intake of 10 per cent. By 1964 the effects of substantial emigration were becoming evident and the 1966 Royal Commission on Medical Education produced an interim report urging immediate expansion of medical education in order to avoid a shortage of doctors. This commission's final report in 1968, known as the Todd Report, recommended a medical school intake target of at least 5000 British medical students a year by 1990. In 1970 the Department of Health and Social Security and the University Grants Committee agreed upon an intake figure for every year of the decade up to 4100 in 1979.

Over the past few years public spending cuts have caused the programme to fall behind schedule and the 4100 target figure has not yet been reached. In 1976 the junior hospital doctors renewed the debate on the realities of the manpower situation since it was felt that Britain was again producing too many doctors. The Junior Hospital Doctors Association consequently advocated a reduction in medical school intake of one-third. The British Medical Association also demanded a freeze on medical school intake. By contrast, the Medical Practitioners Union (1980) has argued, in confirmation of its suggestions in 1976/7, that 34 000 more doctors are needed, as opposed to the mere 25 000 about to be produced by current medical school output. The Union argues that more doctors are required in order to reduce list sizes in general practice to an average of 1750 by the year 2000, to improve the occupational health service, to decasualize general practitioner locum services, to reduce hospital doctors' working hours, and to fill hospital posts in unattractive areas and specialties.

The real problem lies not in absolute numbers, but in defining the role of the doctor and deciding upon the quality of medical care which we should be able to afford. The argument that we will have too many doctors is based on the desire of the medical profession to create more senior posts. In its evidence to the Royal Commission on the National Health Service, the Royal College of Physicians argued that over the past two decades there has been a large increase in the number of junior doctors without a proportionate increase in the number of posts at junior or senior levels. The British Medical Association wants every hospital doctor to have the opportunity of becoming a consultant, and has advocated a substantial increase in the ratio of consultant to junior posts. This should have begun in 1969, when the medical profession and the Department of Health and Social Security agreed that the consultant grade should grow at 4 per cent per annum, and the junior grade by 2½ per cent. However, the expansion of training posts (the annual average between 1968 and 1975 was 5 per cent) has been increasing faster than consultantships (at 4 per cent).

It is possible that there is a danger of unemployment among doctors unless more posts, of all types, are created. This belief is supported by the fact that output from British medical schools is expected to rise from 2600 in 1975 to between 3200 and 3500 by 1981. From this point of view, the issue is not so much whether we have as many doctors as we need, but whether we have as many as we can afford to employ. The Department of Health and Social Security and the University Grants Committee still argue, however, that we need to produce more British doctors in order to reduce the dependence of the National Health Service on foreign-born doctors. At present, 35 per cent of our hospital doctors are both overseas-trained and concentrated in the training grades. Consequently, in 1979 the Royal Commission on the National Health Service reported that the planned output of medical graduates was currently about right and that there is unlikely to be medical unemployment in this country. It was simply felt that doctors would no longer have the wide range of choice of specialty and place of practice that they had been accustomed to. However, a situation of unemployment will not necessarily persuade doctors to practise in less attractive specialties, such as geriatrics or psychiatry, or in less attractive areas, such as the North, Yorkshire, or the West Midlands. Similarly, the recent publication by the Department of Health and Social Security (1978) entitled 'Medical Manpower in the Next Twenty Years' is totally insubstantial as a discussion document: the report weakly argues that it hopes unemployment will not result from present manpower policies.

The Government has altered its opinion about whether we are producing sufficient numbers of doctors every decade since the last war. Why have our medical manpower policies consistently been based on inaccurate predictions? Taking the Willink and Todd Committees, for example – what factors did they fail to consider?

The Willink Committee identified many of the factors included in manpower planning: population size and structure, economic growth, patterns of medical care, doctor–patient ratios, and manpower wastage rates. However, they did not make any assumptions about possible changes in the proportion of resources the Government would allocate to health care, neither did they take into account the possibility that a wealthier country had higher expectations of health care and might wish to devote more resources to it. The committee members used statistics relating to the period 1953 to 1955, while the 1958 official statistics indicated a possible shortage of doctors and a relatively high rate of emigration. One of the main problems of reports on manpower planning is that they are invariably based on outdated figures. As doctors undergo such lengthy training, it is approximately ten years before the implications of policies are realized. There were further shortcomings to the Willink Report. The report overlooked the extension of medical care as a result of progress in medical science. It was also assumed that the population would increase by 4½ per cent from 1955 to 1971. In fact, it had already increased by almost 7½ per cent by 1966. Willink had anticipated that the emigration of doctors would decline. This erroneous judgement, however, was offset by the failure to predict the large increase in the immigration of overseas doctors that has occurred.

The Todd Committee made similar mistakes which have been analysed by Maynard and Walker (1977). The Todd Commissioners made two sets of forecasts – short-term estimates concerned with the 1966 to 1975 period, and long-term estimates concerned with the period 1976 to 1995. Demand for health care was estimated by utilizing arbitrary doctor–patient ratios and staffing ratios. Again, possible policy changes affecting health care were not considered. The predicted supply of doctors was compared with the demand estimate, and policy implications were derived from the result. In their short-term estimate, the Todd Commission underestimated doctor immigration figures and overestimated doctor emigration figures. No account was taken of the number of students who pass Conjoint Board examinations and thus become eligible for registration. Population growth rates were also overestimated, hence the expected shortage of doctors did not occur. The Todd Commission's long-term estimates were similarly based on the incorrect assumptions that there would be a reduction in net emigration and the proportion of female medical graduates would remain constant. The population forecasts used were too high, and their manpower estimates have been affected by the reduction of doctor immigrants due to the effects of the imposition of medical and language proficiency tests after 1975.

What other factors should be considered by planners of medical manpower? Questions should be asked about doctors' career preferences and their potential and existing career structures. The amount of untreated morbidity in the community also requires analysis. How much of it should be actively detected through screening programmes? How many life-saving procedures, such as renal dialysis, should become generally available? How should medical care be organized? How much work at present performed by the doctor could be performed by non-physicians? What is needed is a serious study of the possibilities for the substitution of labour in health care. This issue has been sadly neglected in this country. Even the Department of Health and Social Security's (1978) recent discussion document on medical manpower only makes passing reference to the question of substitution. What is also increasingly needed is a series of alternative manpower forecasts, of the type recently attempted by Maynard and Walker (1978). Finally, any discussion of manpower needs and policies is incomplete without examining the content of the doctor's work.

Workload in general practice

The general practitioner's workload is difficult to assess since it is linked with the concept of quality of care, which is notoriously difficult to define and measure. The number of doctors, list sizes, the distribution of doctors throughout the country, and practice sizes exert only a partial influence on workload. The habits and attitudes of patients, and their use of the health service, as well as the methods of practice and attitudes of doctors, may also influence the quality and nature of general practice.

List size and consultation rates

A basic measure of workload, although crude, is the number of patients registered with each general practitioner. The average list size is approximately 2300 for England and Wales and 2000 for Scotland. These figures have varied little since 1949 (Department of Health and Social Security, Annual Reports 1950–1977; Scottish Home and Health Department, Annual Reports 1960–1977). However, national averages conceal differences between regions. They also ignore differences in workload due to different population age structures and morbidity patterns. South Wales, for example, with an above-average proportion of general practitioners also has a high morbidity rate. The relationship, however, is usually inverse: the greater the morbidity rate, the fewer the resources and health care facilities (Tudor Hart 1971; 1976).

Is there an ideal list size? Many doctors, including the Royal College of General Practitioners, appear to prefer lists of between 2000 and 2500 patients. Little research has been carried out on how many patients a doctor can reasonably be expected to look after. It involves examination of quality care as well as practice organization and manpower. It could be argued that we have a shortage of general practitioners as some doctors have lists in excess of the average figure. However, as other doctors have lists of less than 2300 patients, the problem is partly one of maldistribution. Maldistribution may be a problem only where practices are inefficiently organized. Fry (1972), for example, claims that one doctor can easily care for 3500 patients with no ancillary help. Presumably, with ancillary help doctors could cope with even more patients, while reducing the risk of decreasing the quality of care. An editorial in the *Journal of the Royal College of General Practitioners* (1972) pointed out that in Scandinavia it is common for general practitioners, working within a health team, to care for over 5000 patients each. Marsh and McNay (1974) have shown that when it is possible to work with paramedical staff, doctors can considerably reduce their workload. Certainly, the structural changes in general practice since the 1960s make larger lists more realistic. These changes include the increasing use of appointment systems, the grouping of practices, and the greater use of ancillary staff. Current manpower planning is based on the assumption that the ideal list size is approximately 2500. If doctors can care for more than this number the inference is that we have too many doctors.

It is the doctor's consultation rates, the number of times the patient consults the doctor, which are usually analysed when workload is discussed. Reliable data on such rates are limited. However, it has been pointed out that an international comparison of survey results shows that British doctors see more patients during a one-week period than doctors from other countries (Eimerl and Pearson 1968). Consultation rates are notoriously difficult to compare. A consultation rate is the average number of face-to-face contacts made between doctor and patient during a year and is usually calculated by totalling the number of surgery appointments and home visits. However, such rates depend on definitions and are influenced by the accuracy of recording visits and appointments; the accuracy of the estimate of the practice size; the inclusion or exclusion of figures for immunizations, child care, antenatal care and other clinics; the quality and type of work performed by ancillary staff; and the number of services to temporary residents.

Bearing such problems in mind, what data on consultation rates do exist? Available evidence indicates that the annual surgery consultation rate per patient has been decreasing since 1961 (Howie 1977; Fry 1977). There are several possible explanations for this trend. There has been an expansion of area health authority clinics for antenatal care and child welfare which may have relieved general practitioners of part of their work load. On the other hand, this factor may have been counterbalanced by the changing age and morbidity structure of the population, together with changing expectations about health services. Figures from the Royal College of General Practitioners (1973) also show that there have been 60 per cent reductions in home visiting rates over the past fifty years. This can be partly explained by the changing pattern of disease from acute infections to chronic illness, and partly by the fact that doctors can, to some extent, control their consultation rates. The frequency of doctor-initiated consultations has been shown to be a major factor in contributing to variations in consultations between doctors

(Richardson *et al.* 1973). Existing studies of consultation rates, based on individual practices, have been summarized by Butler (1980). Basically th⸳y show that as list sizes increase, surgery and home consultation rates decrease. For example, practices with list sizes above 3000 had surgery consultation rates of 3.5 or less, whilst most practices with lists below 2500 had consultation rates of 3.0 or more. Similarly, practices with list sizes above 2800 had home consultation rates of 1.0 or less, while those with lists below 2500 had consultation rates in excess of 1.0.

Consultation rates nevertheless remain a crude measure of work load, since they do not take into account the time spent with each patient and on travelling time for home visits. Nor do they measure the content of consultations or examine health needs in terms of medical provision. Activity analyses are seldom performed. What is known is that the average length of the surgery consultation is five to six minutes while the average length of a home visit, including travelling time, is fifteen minutes (Eimerl and Pearson 1968). This is not to ignore the fact that wide regional and individual variations within consultation and length of consultation rates still exist in Britain.

There have also been a number of studies of indirect consultations – consultations by letter, telephone, and by third parties. Wright (1968) revealed a rate of 328 per 1000 patients per annum and Williams (1970) showed an average of ninety indirect consultations per doctor per week. However, indirect consultation rates vary widely between studies (Barber 1971; Morrell and Nicholson 1974).

Additional sources of work about which little is known are telephone messages from other professionals and out of hours calls for home visits. Reedy (1975) has estimated that the rate for telephone calls from other professionals, including hospital calls, per 1000 patients varied between 8.4 and 27.5 during an eight-week period. The rate was inversely related to list size. Even less is known about out of hours calls for home visits, apart from the fact that deputizing services are increasingly being used by doctors to deal with evening, week-end and night work. This is particularly true for doctors practising in urban areas and for those practising alone or in smaller partnerships or groups (Irvine and Jefferys 1971; Cartwright and Anderson 1981).

These rates do not tell us a great deal about the content of the doctor's work or about the quality of care. A limited amount of data do exist which indicate that doctors spend their time performing procedures which could be performed by someone with less training.

This indicates that in terms of the amount of resources devoted to health care, output, or productivity, is low. Studies have shown that complete physical examinations in general practice are rare (Hull 1972; Morrell and Nicholson 1974). Moreover, a recent study suggested that at least 10 per cent of consultations used procedures within the competence of a nurse, and that over half of the total time spent by doctors in consultation with the patient had no clinical component at all (Buchan and Richardson 1973). Doctors' time therefore seems to be spent performing procedures below their level of acquired skill. The activity analysis carried out by Buchan and Richardson showed precisely how time consuming the performance of such procedures is: taking a temperature took almost a minute to record, a vaginal examination took three minutes, a blood test four minutes plus another minute to complete the form, and an ECG took nineteen minutes.

What are the implications of these research findings in terms of future manpower policy and potential workloads? Are more doctors needed in order to reduce list size and make the ten-minute consultation more realistic? This is not the solution if there is an inverse relationship between list size and consultation rate. There are several possible explanations for this relationship, one being that doctors may exert some control over patients' consulting habits. Thus, for example, doctors with large lists would discourage frequent consultations. However, if delegation is practised then larger lists, higher consultation rates, and longer consultation periods per patient could, in theory, be coped with without decreasing the quality of care. Delegation may even increase productivity by making the best use of the doctor's available time in terms of health needs. Whether or not the best use of the doctor's time is made depends on the answer to the question of what the primary health care team is for. In particular, what are general practitioners trained for? The role of the general practitioner needs defining before the issue of manpower can be satisfactorily explored.

There is undoubtedly a need for producing more ancillary staff to enable doctors to concentrate on their medical skills. At a time of threatened doctor unemployment, a situation likely to be worsened as the Professional and Linguistic Assessment Board's tests for immigrant doctors have been relaxed for EEC doctors, a policy of maximum delegation is not likely to be viewed favourably by the medical profession. On the other hand, a situation of doctor unemployment does not necessarily resolve the problem of too few general practitioners in unattractive areas. Nor is it an excuse for doctors to perform tasks below their level of skill. The future of primary health care demands a clear definition of the roles of health care professionals and the efficient use of ancillary personnel. Even in terms of the current work of the general practitioner, and in terms of current available manpower, there is a need for further delegation.

5

DELEGATION IN GENERAL PRACTICE: ADVANTAGES AND DISADVANTAGES

Cost–benefit analyses

The doctor is a highly trained person. The production of a medical student is also expensive. The five-year medical-school training costs approximately £40000 per student. As the doctor's time is such a valuable commodity, greater delegation of routine medical procedures to non-physicians might result in financial economies as well as greater efficiency. However, few adequate cost–benefit analyses of the concept of the physician's assistant or of the expanded nurse role exist. On the one hand it might be argued that delegation to non-physicians is not cost-effective, because this increases the demand for health care. That the employment of ancillary staff generates an increased demand, and consequently an increase in provision, in health services has already been demonstrated (Bailit *et al.* 1975). This leads to an increase in health care costs, unless the result is that patients' conditions are seen earlier than they otherwise would be and are hence less difficult and costly to treat. Costs may be further increased because consultations with non-physicians such as nurse practitioners are apparently longer than consultations with doctors (Bessman 1974). However, if a main part of the nurse practitioner's role is, for example, to promote health by giving health education then, in the long run, such a system may be cost-effective. Even if it is not, this is not necessarily a disadvantage. Beck (1971), for example, has argued that the high cost of our present method of organization is the least desirable of the arguments upon which to base a programme of further delegation. The implication of such an argument is that delegation is desirable only because it is cheaper than the 'real thing'. It is, on the other hand, incumbent upon advocates of delegation to demonstrate that the arguably less expensive resource provides health care of equal or better quality.

Productivity

Contradictory statements are to be found in the literature concerning the productivity resulting from delegation. Although no significant differences have emerged indicating increased productivity in the United States since the introduction of physicians' assistants or nurse practitioners, physicians are sometimes said to feel their own productivity has increased (Smith 1974). However, computer simulation of general practice in Canada has shown that the addition of a nurse does not necessarily result in increased practice efficiency, economy, or a saving of the doctor's time. This was found to be the case because improvements in practice efficiency as a consequence of the employment of a nurse depended on factors such as the ratio of physicians to nurses, the ratio of rooms to personnel employed, the duties of the nurse, the type of responsibilities delegated, and the use and type of appointment system. A nurse or physician's assistant cannot be expected to increase physician efficiency, effectiveness, or economy if placed in a practice with few facilities and little practice organization (Sagar, Morrow, and Lees 1972).

What are the effects of delegation on productivity in British general practice? Results from studies in Britain during the 1960s were equivocal in their estimates of the time-saving abilities of the nurse. The Royal College of General Practitioners (1968) reported an experiment in the employment of nurses in four general practices in the North-East of England. It was found that the use of a nurse resulted in a gradual fall in annual doctor–patient consultation rates as the number of services performed by the nurse increased. Not only was a saving of the doctors' time effected, but doctors also made more accurate clinical predictions during this period and experienced more satisfaction with their work. However, Hodgkin and Gillie (1968), commenting on their practices in the same report, found that contrary to expectations the nurse actually saved the doctors little time. One reason given for this was the operation of Parkinson's Law: the tendency to unconsciously utilize time saved. For example, more time was spent with elderly patients and on home visits. In this sense, delegation increased productivity, at least in the crude sense of the term as the content of the consultations is unknown.

Hasler and his colleagues (1968) showed that nurses attached to their group practice had, by performing delegated medical tasks, enabled the doctor to spend more time with each patient. Kuenssberg (1971) found that the employment of nurses in his practice resulted in the practice of more thorough clinical medicine. Attention was paid to history taking, the use of diagnostic instruments, physical examinations, and the taking of specimens for laboratory analysis; simple referrals to hospitals decreased. Delegation may not reduce the doctor's workload simply because higher standards of care are then, hopefully, provided. Again, Cartwright and Anderson (1981) found that doctors with privately employed nurses – nurses working in treatment rooms – more often felt that their nurses frequently did things the doctor would do if there was no nurse. Seventy-five per cent of those with an employed nurse felt this in comparison with 45 per cent of other doctors. They also found that doctors with an attached or employed nurse were more likely to carry out procedures such as fitting intrauterine devices, excising cysts, taking blood, stitching cuts, and examining the vagina with a speculum, than were doctors without a nurse. They found that nurses were more likely to undertake a procedure if the doctor also did it, and vice versa. This is possibly because doctors and nurses are both frequently involved in the procedure at the same time, the nurse acting in an assisting capacity. Such an arrangement appears wasteful of manpower resources if the nurse is capable of performing any of these procedures alone.

Quality of care

How likely is it that the quality of care would suffer as a result of a policy of discouraging the performance of routine medical procedures by those with the highest medical skills and qualifications possible? It often appears to be assumed that the ideal way to deliver health care is through the services of excellently trained physicians and that any other method is second best. It is possible, however, that non-physicians may perform certain tasks better than a doctor. Doctors may become bored when performing routine tasks such as ear syringing or venepuncture and thus may not perform them very well. Non-physicians, having more patience because of their different backgrounds, may perform them with more care. Delegation will also free the doctor to concentrate on more complex medical skills and to spend more time with each patient. However, Cartwright and Anderson (1981) found that patients did not think their doctor was better at examining them thoroughly if he or she worked with a nurse. On the other hand, working with a nurse does not necessarily imply that delegation is being practised efficiently. The fact that doctors in these authors' sample also performed the tasks they delegated suggests that it is not. This may explain why doctors without a nurse were no less likely to enjoy their work than those with one.

Although there are no studies linking good quality care and delegation in Britain, studies in the United States and Canada have provided positive evidence. For example, Spitzer and his colleagues (1974) conducted a randomized trial testing the competence of the nurse practitioner as the initial contact in the surgery in comparison with the doctor. They concluded that a nurse practitioner can provide such care as safely and effectively, with as much satisfaction to patients, as a doctor. The nurse was able to work alone in 67 per cent of all patient consultations. This study prompted *The Lancet* (1974) to ask whether British doctors are currently over-trained for their work. The point is not that general practitioners are not needed, or are over-trained, but that they need the collaboration of other health workers so that they can concentrate on the medical skills in which they were trained.

Komaroff and his colleagues (1974) have also evaluated the performance of physicians' assistants acting as the initial contact for patients by using problem-oriented protocols in the management of patients with diabetes and hypertension. The protocols directed the assistants in determining what data to collect, and whether or not the patient needed to be referred to the physician. Physicians judged the assistants to be competent at history taking and physical examination. Protocols were said to have been used successfully because relatively few conditions accounted for the majority of out-patient visits. Thus, the development of protocols for the most common conditions may have a relatively large impact on decreasing the doctor's workload.

Spector and his colleagues attempted to evaluate the quality of medical care provided by trained nurses in an internal medical clinic. These nurses performed various technical procedures which had once been regarded as duties of the physician and followed up patients seen by the physician. Physicians judged the nurses' performance as adequate and physician consultations decreased during the experimental period whilst nurse–patient contacts increased (Spector *et al.* 1975).

In the same year Bailit and his associates (1975) found that nurse practitioners could make diagnostic assessments and manage patients in well-child and minor illness situations as effectively as the doctor. There are a number of studies indicating that non-physicians can safely screen patients and perform many technical medical tasks. However, unwarranted generalizations from favourable evaluation studies should be avoided. Existing studies typically evaluate the performance of only one or two nurses or assistants who may not be representative. Moreover, there is no consistent opinion of how to measure quality of care. The outcome of treatment cannot be adequately measured in short-term studies.

What about quality of care from the point of view of the patient? It is possible that patients might not find nurses, or any other type of auxiliary worker, acceptable substitutes for the doctor in many situations. Such personnel may be perceived as forming a barrier between patient and doctor, an accusation levelled against receptionists on occasions (Williams 1977). A system of further delegation should only be operated with the patient's consent, and access to the doctor should never be denied. In any case, the assumption that no third party should intervene between doctor and patient is questionable, especially with the increasing complexity of medical care. Studies of patient satisfaction with treatment or assessment by a nurse, moreover, yield largely positive results. The first attempt to measure patients' responses to the introduction of a nurse in general practice was the study by Smith and Mottram (1967). The majority of patients approved of nurses, found them helpful, and regarded the system as satisfactory. An extension of this study confirmed these results (Smith and O'Donovan 1970). Both studies were based on the practice of a nurse undertaking initial home visits to assess whether a doctor's visit was necessary.

On the other hand, a study of patients in one general practice found that, although three-quarters of respondents felt that nurses were an important aid to the doctor, only half felt they were an important aid for the patient. The majority agreed that nurses should perform technical treatments, such as injections, although only half felt it was a good idea for nurses to see patients initially in the surgery to decide whether a doctor's examination was necessary. Few patients were in favour of nurses performing initial home visits (Cunningham, Bevan, and Floyd 1972). However, patients who had experienced contact with nurses held more favourable attitudes on these measures. Working-class people appeared to value them most. This may be because these people have a less satisfactory relationship with their doctors, as Cartwright and O'Brien (1976) have found. On the other hand, many respondents felt the nurse could be valuable in giving confidence to patients and two-thirds had experienced no difficulties in talking to the nurse.

A larger survey of 3100 patients in one practice by Marsh and Kaim Caudle (1976) found that half the patients questioned said they would not mind if a nurse visited them if they had sent for the doctor. Three-quarters of those who had received such initial visits from the nurse were satisfied with the advice and treatment given. However, more than half would still have preferred a visit from the doctor. Again, objections were more frequent among those who had not experienced this method of organization than among those who had. The majority of those who had received clinical treatments from the nurse (injections, taking blood, ear syringing, blood pressure), after they had seen the doctor, were satisfied with the treatment. However, one in five respondents objected to a nurse treating minor complaints (skin rash, septic skin, earache) in place of a doctor. As the authors concluded, people tend to have a preference for the familiar, thus in unfamiliar situations good communications are essential. The authors also felt that the relevant training of nurses in this branch of health care would enhance patient satisfaction.

More encouraging results were established by Cartwright and Anderson (1981). They found that three-quarters of their national random sample of patients felt it was an advantage from the patient's point of view when the doctor had a nurse working at the surgery. Once again, favourable attitudes were linked to contact with a nurse, or at least knowledge of a nurse in the practice. Unfortunately, patients were not asked for their views of nurses performing tasks in the place of a doctor.

Similarly, patient satisfaction surveys in the United States have found that patients without experience of treatment from non-physicians lack confidence in their ability (Litman 1972), whereas patients who have received treatment from such personnel as physicians' assistants and nurse practitioners are satisfied and find them competent. Such favourable attitudes have been found by Nelson (1974) and Komaroff (1974) and their colleagues. In fact, patients' attitudes to care given by nurse practitioners have revealed a higher degree of satisfaction than have their attitudes towards care given by doctors (Linn 1976). There is also evidence of more patient compliance with treatments prescribed by nurses than those prescribed by doctors. This is possibly because of longer consultation periods with nurses, in comparison with doctors, or because of the reduced status gap between patient and professional (Fairweather and Kifolo 1972; Bessman 1974).

Legal responsibility

The trend in Britain whereby nurses have become increasingly involved in the performance of procedures which have traditionally been medical responsibilities has led to uncertainties over their legal position. Until these have been resolved it may not be practical to recommend further delegation.

General practitioners were empowered to delegate tasks to nurses in 1966 when the terms of service under the National Health Service Acts were revised. As a result, there are no legal constraints in this country to prevent the delegation of clinical and diagnostic duties to a nurse or other health worker. The only exception is prescription writing which, in theory, can be performed only by physicians – apart from occupational health nurses in certain circumstances. Despite the 1966 Act, many professionals seem unsure of the position of the doctor and nurse where delegation is concerned. These uncertainties have led to the publication of numerous guidelines by the Department of Health and Social Security and by various professional bodies. Statements issued by the Medical Defence Union (1970) and the Queen's Institute of District Nursing (1970) indicated that the doctor is responsible for any negligence on the part of the nurse when the latter is acting in the doctor's presence, carrying out the doctor's treatment, and when under the doctor's direct supervision. However, when the nurse is performing delegated duties and when the doctor allows the nurse to perform these in his or her own way, then the nurse is liable for personal acts of negligence. Such statements may appear confusing for practitioners. For example, where nurses act on their own initiative, this may not be the direct result of any formal policy on the part of the doctors, but a method of practice which may simply have evolved in an unsystematic way. While doctors who work with nurses should be encouraged to formulate a policy concerning delegation, there is no guarantee that they will do so. Further guidelines have recently been issued by the Department of Health and Social Security (1977b) in their Health Circular. This states that in an action for damages a nurse may be held legally liable if he or she has failed to exercise skills properly expected, or if the nurse has undertaken tasks he or she is not competent to perform. The doctor, it was stated, may be held guilty of negligence if it is shown that authority was conferred on a nurse to perform a task outside the scope of his or her normal duties, or for which he or she had no special qualification.

Delegation was approved of only when the following conditions were satisfied: the nurse has been trained for the performance of the task and agrees to undertake it, this training is professionally recognized in addition to being recognized by the employing authorities, both the employing authorities and the professions recognize the task as suitable for delegation, and the delegating doctor has been assured of the competence of the nurse. These guidelines reinforce the views of the Royal College of Nursing as expressed in their 1978 report on the position of the nurse. The Department of Health and Social Security also recommended that delegation should be practised within the context of a clearly defined policy, based on discussion and agreement between those responsible for providing medical and nursing services. Although official policy recommends that such discussion should take place at local levels, variations in national patterns of delegation do little to resolve the legal confusion existing in this area. For example in 1971, the Department of Health sanctioned the delegation of vaccination against smallpox to nurses. In 1976, however, due to continuing confusion over legal responsibility and the variety of codes of practice in operation by different area health authorities, the Department again issued guidelines on the delegation of vaccination and immunization (Department of Health and Social Security 1971; 1976b). The Department still refused to recommend that a national code of practice be adopted. While guidelines on the issue of delegation may be scrutinized by area health authorities, there is no guarantee that individual general practitioners will give them careful consideration.

The literature on the practice organization of individual general practitioners illustrates how the degree of autonomy allowed the nurse by the doctor varies considerably. Some doctors draw up rules for the practice of delegation, such as the insistence that the nurse does not give advice, and on methods of reporting back the patient's condition and treatment to the doctor (Hodgkin 1967). Others allow the nurse more freedom to use personal initiative (Smith and Mottram 1967). While nurses may be capable of making assessments and of performing a wide range of medical procedures, until uniform training courses in treatment room work are available to all nurses, it is likely that the confusion surrounding legal responsibility will continue. In the case of privately employed practice nurses, for example, the only training they are likely to receive in performing delegated tasks is that given by the doctors employing them, although some area health authorities now offer these nurses instruction. Thus, those nurses most likely to perform medical tasks have not necessarily received adequate training.

Practice nurses employed by general practitioners appear isolated due to their lack of recognition and identity. The fault is partly their own. For example, Reedy and his colleagues found that 44 per cent of employed nurses were members of either the Royal College of Nursing or of a trade union (Reedy *et al.* 1980a). In recognition of their professional isolation, practice nurses in some areas have formed practice nurses' associations. These bodies have approached local schools of nursing and have, as a result, been given study day invitations. They have also been given permission by hospital consultants to attend their clinics to learn new techniques and procedures. The Royal College of Nursing has also begun to organize study days for practice nurses (Wrightson 1975). In addition, in 1971 a discussion group course for treatment room nurses was organised by the Thames Valley Faculty of the Royal College of General Practitioners (Hasler *et al.* 1972). A subcommittee of the East Anglia Faculty of the Royal College of General Practitioners has designed a training course for practice nurses. The skills of the practice nurse have been defined and the educational objectives of this course have been described by Mourin (1980). However, training schemes for practice nurses are still at the experimental stage. Although a programme of specialized nurse training in this area has been called for by the Royal College of Nursing and the Royal College of General Practitioners in their Joint Report (1974), the Joint Board for Clinical Nursing Studies (1978) has rejected a course under its aegis. The Board argued that since the nature of tasks delegated to nurses and the extent of delegation will vary considerably from area to area, training should be provided on a local rather than on a national basis.

The Royal College of Nursing (1977) has pointed to the additional problems which are created by the dual employment of nurses by the area health authority and by the general practitioner. The privately employed nurse is accountable to the doctor. On the other hand, attached nursing staff, employed by the area health authority, are accountable to a nursing officer. The Royal College of Nursing believes that this dual situation leads to the anomalous position in which some members of the team do not possess professional autonomy. The privately employed practice, or treatment room, nurse, for example, is not accountable to another nurse, as are area health authority employed nurses, but to a member of another profession. The Royal College sees this situation leading to further legal problems. For example, legally, the duties of the nurse employed by the area health authority cannot be arbitrarily extended by the doctor. However, the doctor may not always realize this and may suggest that such nurses undertake medical tasks outside the scope of their role as defined by the authority. This limitation, of course, is the reason why some doctors employ their own nurses. For example, Waters, Sandeman, and Lunn (1980) argue that they delegated many tasks to their own practice nurse, so enabling her to make an important contribution to the work of the practice, which they would have been unable to do if they relied on attached nurses requiring area health authority authorization.

So much uncertainty appears to exist over the delegation of minor clinical procedures that little attention has been paid to more complex types of delegation. It is doubtful whether progress will be made towards resolving legal uncertainties unless uniform training courses for nurses undertaking extended roles are systematically instituted. Moreover, until nurses are uniformly trained in medical procedures which could be delegated they are not likely to become nursing procedures in their own right. Consequently, the controversy over whether nurses should perform these tasks will persist, and patterns of delegation will continue to vary.

Perhaps the main problem is the controversy within nursing itself, over whether it is in the professional interests of nursing to perform procedures within the domain of another profession. Until the nursing profession decides whether it wishes nurses to undertake certain medical tasks in a systematic fashion, it is doubtful whether these procedures will ever be incorporated in basic or post-basic nurse training courses on a national basis. Perhaps the most recent example of this controversy is the issue of the legality and desirability of nurses carrying out medically induced abortions. The Department of Health believes that, providing a doctor decides on an abortion, he or she does not have to perform every action in the procedure. This judgment has been upheld by a high-court judge. However, the Royal College of Nursing has objected that nurses are not legally insured to perform such abortions (*Nursing Mirror* 1980). Basically, legal problems are being used partly as a camouflage for the College's real concern over the proper role of the nurse.

Little guidance on legal issues can be found in the situation in the United States. Unlike in Britain, definitions of medicine are made at state level. This leads to complexity when there are approximately fifty different states involved. Legally, it is generally held that no one except a licensed physician should diagnose, treat, operate, or prescribe. However, United States law does accept two basic concepts: custom and usage and standing orders (Sadler 1974). These permit physicians to define their terms of practice themselves in certain settings. In theory, this avoids the problem of having to change various aspects of the law relating to the practice of medicine to meet changing situations. Many states still felt the necessity to pass new legislation before delegation to physicians' assistants or nurse practitioners could be practised. By 1975, thirty-seven states had passed such legislation relating to these new health practitioners.

However, the legal position of the nurse practitioner, as opposed to a physician's assistant, is still not easily defined. Unlike physicians' assistants, who need licensure before they can practise, the initial nursing qualifications possessed by nurse practitioners enables them to make nursing decisions and to prescribe and perform treatments independently of the physician. Debate continues over whether the functions of the nurse practitioner come within the scope of the Nurse Practice Act without need for amendment. As Reedy (1978) has pointed out, this is still an unresolved issue. There is a fear that the utilization of intermediate health practitioners will increase malpractice claims. Sadler, Sadler, and Bliss (1974) have argued, on the other hand, that such personnel should reduce malpractice suits. For example, the effective utilization of such assistants should allow the physician to concentrate on those medical procedures and decisions for which he or she has been trained. These authors also claim that a malpractice suit often results from poor doctor–patient rapport rather than negligence. Long waiting periods and hurried consultations may produce patient dissatisfaction. However, it has been shown that when a physician's assistant is employed patients' waiting times are reduced and they receive more attention (Elliot Dixon 1970; Pondy 1970). Moreover, as Reedy (1978) has pointed out, no malpractice claims against such personnel are known to exist.

Would doctors delegate?

Even if it is decided that a more extensive degree of delegation to either further-trained nurses or to physicians' assistants would be advantageous in Britain, the successful introduction of such personnel will depend on the willingness of existing professionals to work with them. For example, if doctors have a vested interest in maintaining their professional control only minor organizational innovations may be accepted. The degree to which doctors seek to exert professional control and dominance over other health occupations partly depends on the degree of threat they perceive from them. Furthermore, as role changes within one occupation, for example, nursing, will inevitably have repercussions on related occupations, such as medicine, and vice versa, then conflict may be inevitable.

It was previously argued that the role and status of the British general practitioner is still uncertain. Until the role of the general practitioner has been clearly defined, and until the status of general practice is more secure, doctors may be reluctant to delegate any more of their medical functions for fear of further uncertainties. They may also be reluctant to work with new types of health practitioners due to these very feelings of role and status threat. Merely to inform the medical profession that the further delegation of clinical and diagnostic procedures to trained personnel may result in increased efficiency in health care is unlikely to make them receptive towards such innovation. Where general practice is concerned, it will be of little avail to inform doctors that delegation will enable them to concentrate on their unique skills if no accepted definition of these skills exists. Several attitude studies, based on doctors in the United States, support these statements. Unfortunately, most are weakened by low response rates and all are based on postal questionnaires.

For example, Heiman and Dempsey (1976) investigated doctors' and nurses' attitudes towards the nurse practitioner. They found that a critical issue in defining the extent of an expanded nurse role was not nurses' capabilities but the attitudes of both nurses and physicians towards allowing a nurse independence and power in decision making. Professional interests appeared to intervene with the effect that the scope of the nurse's role would be limited. In a similar study, Reed and Roghmann (1971) found that medical students and house physicians were hostile towards the concept of an expanded role for the nurse. On the other hand, nurses themselves were more receptive towards the concept. This finding was supported by a smaller scale study by McCormack and Crawford (1971).

While studies in the United States have found that many physicians feel they need help with various routine procedures such as medical history taking, cervical smears and children's physical examinations, few would be inclined to employ additional help in their own practices if it were available. For example, Riddick (1971) and Yankauer (1968) and their colleagues found that while about 60 per cent of doctors may believe that such help is needed, only 30 per cent would have employed help. Similarly, Coy and Hansen (1969) found that almost two-thirds of their sample of physicians believed that physicians' assistants were needed, but less than half said they would use such personnel in their own practices. It was also found that, in practice, respondents would delegate little responsibility to such assistants. Some doctors were willing to delegate simpler procedures but not procedures which approached the domain of their specialty skills. Over two-thirds of doctors would confine an assistant to the performance of technical procedures, such as intravenous injections and catheterizations. Less than a fifth were in favour of assistants performing physical examinations, although almost two-thirds were in favour of them taking a medical history. Similarly, Borland (1972) found that doctors considered that activities involving the formulation of a diagnosis or prescription of a course of treatment were the least appropriate duties for assistants, whereas routine clinical tests, for example laboratory tests, were considered to be the most appropriate duties. Again, Lawrence and his colleagues (1977) found that only one-third of their respondents would employ a nurse practitioner, whereas over half approved of the concept but would not hire one. Similar attitudes were expressed towards a physician's assistant. These findings were confirmed by Fottler and his colleagues (1978) who also found that doctors who already employed a nurse, doctors in group practices and more recent medical graduates were the most receptive towards the concept of delegation.

Eichenberger and his colleagues initially presented more optimistic results. They found that 46 per cent of doctors held favourable attitudes towards a physician's assistant performing a complete medical examination, although 9 per cent placed restrictions on this; 82 per cent were in favour of an assistant taking a medical history, although 43 per cent placed restrictions on this; 52 per cent were in favour of a physician's assistant making a preliminary judgement or diagnosis, whilst 24 per cent placed restrictions on this. Thus, favourable attitudes camouflage many reservations and should be viewed with caution. These authors found that general practitioners were more hostile than specialists towards the concept of a physician's assistant, generally claiming that there was no need for such personnel. These doctors are perhaps most likely to perceive more role overlap with such assistants and, hence, most role threat (Eichenberger *et al.* 1970). The discovery that less recent medical graduates held least favourable attitudes towards such assistance may be explained in terms of the conservatism of such doctors. A stronger degree of conservatism among such doctors may be expected, a conservatism which is enhanced by their middle-class backgrounds and training and ossified with age (Fottler, Gibson, and Pinchoff 1978). Certainly, Mechanic (1974), in his study of physicians' attitudes towards innovation, found conservatism to be related to lack of receptivity towards physicians' assistants, at least among doctors not practising in groups. Moreover, these doctors are generally those who are older. Among non-group practitioners, Mechanic also found a relationship between receptivity towards physicians' assistants and the possession of a broader conception of the physician's role. These doctors may feel less threatened by delegation as they tend to possess specialist qualifications and were thus less likely to be interested in simple, routine procedures.

Less is known about the reactions of British doctors towards the concept of delegation and those of the nurse practitioner and physician's assistant. Apart from a recent survey by Miller and Backett (1980) on doctors' attitudes towards an extended role for the nurse, all that exist are a few studies of doctors' attitudes towards attached nursing staff, and towards the delegation of very minor procedures. None of these studies are very informative. We do know, of course, that the attachment of nurses to general practices is now widespread, and doctors are also increasingly employing their own nurses (Reedy, Philips, and Newell 1976). However, surveys in the mid-1960s, when attachment schemes were in their initial stages, revealed that general practitioners' attitudes towards them were mixed (Wessex Regional Hospital Board 1964). Abel (1969) found that one reason for the failure of attachment schemes was the indifference of doctors towards them. A small survey by Hockey (1968) revealed that general practitioners possessed quite mixed reactions to the notion of nurses carrying out initial home visits for assessment purposes. More favourable results were presented by Boddy (1969) in a random survey of Scottish general practitioners. He found that the majority of practitioners questioned were willing to delegate medical procedures to a nurse. However, Boddy's questions related to simple procedures such as injections, dressings, bathing and giving enemas. A recent postal survey of 533 randomly selected general practitioners found that two-thirds of doctors were in favour of an expanded role for treatment room nurses and were prepared to delegate clinical tasks to a nurse. These doctors tended to be aged under fifty and to hold regular meetings with other members of the practice. However, included in their figure of two-thirds of doctors in favour are 14 per cent who see only a temporary place for such nurses while there is a shortage of general practitioners. Altogether, just 45 per cent saw a permanent place for them. Unfortunately, the authors questioned doctors about the tasks to be delegated collectively, rather than individually. For example, they asked about history taking, examination, diagnosis, and advice on treatment all in the same question. Thus, they do not have any data on doctors' opinions on the possibilities for delegating each individual task (Miller and Backett 1980).

So how willing might doctors be in the future to further extend delegation? What are the main factors inhibiting the transfer of functions from doctors to other health care workers? Studies have shown that older doctors, practising alone or from smaller groups of two or three, are least likely to introduce innovations into their practices (Irvine and Jefferys 1971; Cartwright and Anderson 1981). The previously cited studies of doctors' attitudes towards delegation in the United States confirm this. Will attitudes change as younger doctors enter general practice? Miller and Backett's research indicates that they might. However, attitudes will not necessarily change as the medical profession has the power to reproduce its own structure. This can be seen in the selection and training of medical students and the career and staffing structure of doctors following qualification. The profession controls entry into medical schools, and is thus able to select entrants who are likely to conform to established norms and values. In addition, large numbers of entrants come from social classes one and two and have at least one parent who is medically qualified (Report of the Royal Commission on Medical Education 1968; Robson 1973). Medical education is also a process by which the medical culture is reinforced. The resulting consensus may act to deter the delegation of professional responsibilities to non-physicians who have not participated in this socialization process. Before widespread delegation can occur, doctors need to be taught to delegate. Such training demands teachers committed to the concept of team care. There is no certainty that such teachers exist in sufficient numbers to overcome the conservatism inherent in the system. Indeed, undergraduate training in general practice itself is notoriously poor.

Rigid adherence to concepts of independence and autonomy may also be responsible for the reluctance of physicians to practise delegation. Physicians have traditionally assumed command, made decisions, and shouldered responsibilities and will, not unexpectedly, be reluctant to share these functions. This reluctance may be linked to conservatism, and if roles are insecure, as in the case of general practitioners, this reluctance may be reinforced. Although doctors may perceive delegation as a surrender of power, this is not necessarily what happens. As Reedy (1972) has pointed out, delegation should enhance the responsibility of the delegator as it coincides with the concept of final medical responsibility.

It has already been pointed out that older doctors possess the most conservative attitudes and this may explain the relationship between older doctors and single-handed or small group practice (Cartwright and Anderson 1981). This being the case, there is little point in encouraging delegation until some of the features of the present organization of general practice have been eroded. The concept of an expanded role for the nurse, or of a physician's assistant, is not logical in a country where single-handed and small group practice predominate. There is no future for the reallocation of tasks within the health team if no health team exists. Furthermore, about a quarter of doctors not practising from a health centre have no treatment room (Cartwright and Anderson 1981). Similarly, Reedy, Metcalfe, de Roumani, and Newell (1980b) found that one-fifth of the attached nurses questioned in their survey had nowhere to treat patients and resorted to expedients such as treating them in premises belonging to other practitioners. As younger doctors enter general practice its structure may change. However, as previously argued, even younger doctors have received some socialization in the values of the previous generation of doctors.

Furthermore, in contrast with hospital doctors and with the consultant at the apex of the hierarchy of medical and paramedical staff, independence appears to have been traditionally interpreted by doctors in general practice as single-handed practice with little ancillary help. Single-handed practice may therefore be a reflection of a practitioner's desire for this narrowly defined conception of independence. Teamwork may be regarded as alien. Unlike the consultant, the general practitioner has no secure role at the apex of a hierarchy of staff and there is little incentive for doctors adhering to rigid notions of independence to change. In fact, debate exists over who, if anyone, should lead the primary health care team, a debate which must make the general practitioner feel further threatened.

The controversy over delegation, which has not yet developed in Britain as extensively as in other countries, is but one facet of the struggle to maintain professional dominance. Paramedical groups are currently attempting to obtain greater control over their practices, and to initiate and carry out their own unique professional responsibilities. Psychiatrists, in particular, are experiencing role conflicts with psychologists and psychiatric nurses. Autonomy of action is a crucial factor in the dominance of the medical profession. Decision making, such as that involved in being the professional of first contact, may be regarded as part of the autonomy of the profession. Thus, attempts to encourage doctors to practise extensive delegation, and especially the delegation of initial assessments, may be seen as professionally threatening. In view of such conflicts and threats, together with a possible fear on the part of doctors that medicine may become demystified with delegation, the resistance of many doctors to the concept of further delegation may be expected (Bowling 1980a; 1980c).

The extent of delegation today

How widespread is the delegation of medical procedures to ancillary staff in general practice? As we have already seen, area health authority employed community nurses appear to be transferring more of their work from patients' homes to general practitioners' surgeries. This practice saves the nurse's travelling time, although it is only possible when patients are mobile. Doctors are also increasingly employing their own surgery nurses. According to Reedy, Philips, and Newell (1976) the number of such nurses in 1974 was 3100. In relation to the total number of general practitioners this figure is small. Moreover, Reedy *et al.* (1980b) found that employed nurses only work approximately twenty-three hours a week, most of this time being spent in the surgery. Although the attached nurses employed by the area health authority to work in the community worked thirty-nine hours a week, only 18 per cent spent more than two hours a week in the practice premises. It is difficult to see how teamwork and further delegation can be encouraged in this situation.

Weisz (1972), on the basis of an international literature survey, found the following tasks to be the most commonly delegated:

refractory
visual field test
measurement of intraocular tension
hearing tests
otoscopy
gynaecological cytology
history taking
complete physical examination
intravenous injection
episiotomy
suturing of a perineal rupture
vacuum extraction
defibrillation
introduction of gastric tube
suturing of laceration
operation for entropion
operation for cataract

intravenous infusion
application of plaster casts
insertion of IUDs
condensing and carving amalgram
restorations
closed-chest cardiac massage
mouth-to-mouth breathing

Of course, many of these procedures do not come within the scope of primary care in the United Kingdom. Unfortunately, very little is known about the extent and type of delegation in British general practice. On the basis of a survey of the literature in this country, Reedy (1972) has listed those tasks which have been recorded as being performed by nurses working in general practice over the past twenty years or so. This reveals the performance of a much simpler type of procedure than those listed by Weisz, partly reflecting the less technical nature of general practice in comparison with hospital medicine:

height and weight measurement
temperature, pulse and respiration rate recording
blood pressure recording
chemical testing of urine and faeces
supervising the collection of urine and faeces for the laboratory
bacteriological sampling for transmission to the laboratory
estimation of ESR and haemoglobin within the practice
venepuncture
immunology performance of Planotest
performance of cervical smears
electrocardiography
audiometry
tonometry
use of peak flow meter and vitalograph
reception and assessment of patients attending without appointments
initial home visits
revisits
routine visiting of chronic sick
surgical dressings
insertion of sutures
removal of sutures
incision of boils and abscesses
aspiration of cysts
therapeutic injections (subcutaneous and intramuscular)
ear syringing and other aural treatments and dressings
application of plasters and cervical collars
application of splints

changing vaginal pessaries
simple physiotherapy
counselling
supervision of certain types of patient
dietary supervision
advising receptionists over patients' needs
chaperoning
preparation of patients for doctor and assisting at examination or treatment
liaison with hospital in-patients and laboratory
maintenance and care of equipment, dressings, drugs and linen
supervision of sterilization and antisepsis procedures
transport of patients to and from surgery
immunizations and vaccinations (including smallpox)
skin testing for allergy
desensitizing injections
teaching patients illness management and hygiene
supervision of certain clinics
dispensing in rural practices

From this list it does appear that nurses may have quite an extensive role in general practice already. However, as most studies have been based on individual practices, which are probably unrepresentative, little is still known about the prevalence or regularity of delegation in general practice. A recent national study of nursing activities in primary care (Reedy *et al.* 1980b) has shown that area health authority attached nurses score highly in the performance of caring activities, such as bed bathing, feeding and toileting patients. General practitioner employed nurses scored highly in the performance of technical procedures, such as venepuncture, ear syringing and incision of boils. However, nurses were simply asked whether they had ever done these things, amongst others, during their present employment or attachment and during the last month. In the case of each procedure listed, fewer, sometimes considerably fewer, of the nurses had performed the task in the last month. Unfortunately the frequency, or regularity, with which nurses performed the tasks was not measured. Similarly, Cartwright and Anderson (1981) asked their national sample of general practitioners whether their nurses ever undertook procedures such as ear syringing, venepuncture, suturing, incision of abscesses, excision of cysts, fitting of IUDs or assisting at vaginal examinations. The proportion of employed nurses performing ear syringing, assisting at vaginal examinations, and taking blood was found to be 93 per cent, 80 per cent and 57 per cent respectively. The respective proportions for attached nurses were 73 per cent, 53 per cent, and 45 per cent. Far fewer nurses were found to perform suturing, incision of abscesses, excision of cysts or fitting of IUDs. The proportion of employed nurses performing these procedures was 28 per cent, 26 per cent, 3 per cent, and 2 per cent respectively. Again, the respective proportions for attached nurses were 14 per cent, 6 per cent, 1 per cent and none of the attached nurses ever fitted IUDs. Since no measure of frequency was used, all that we know from such studies is that the more complex the task, the less likely the nurse is, especially in the case of attached nurses, to perform it.

The delegation of initial home visiting may be a further area in which the efficiency of primary care can be increased and which may also result in a better utilization of skills. Patients request home visits in preference to visiting a doctor for several reasons, for the severity of the illness is not necessarily the determining factor. Previous experience of illness may influence the patient's reactions to symptoms and determine subsequent behaviour. The distance a person lives from the surgery, the availability of convenient transport, the existence of children to look after, or weather conditions may all affect the number of requests for home visits. If the fundamental reason for a number of home visits is not the severity of the illness, there is a strong case in favour of another member of the practice, for example a nurse, dealing with them. However, the delegation of initial home visits for assessment or diagnostic purposes is a controversial issue. Just one in eight of those doctors with a nurse in Cartwright and Anderson's (1981) study felt it was appropriate for a nurse to make such first contacts in patients' homes. This attitude is not consistent with the fact that revisits are not made for a high percentage of acute new calls – the implication being that many of these calls are for minor conditions (Hicks 1976).

Nurses could be taught to recognize infectious diseases and make a decision about whether the doctor needs to make an immediate visit or even whether the doctor needs to make a visit at all. Marsh (1969) found that a nurse could quite safely undertake many of his chronic visits as well as many of his follow-up visits to acutely ill patients. Smith and Mottram (1967) and Smith and O'Donovan (1970) have demonstrated that a nurse can effectively act as a diagnostician and therapist in the home. Smith and O'Donovan even found that a nurse could carry out 60 per cent of all initial home visits, and that only in one in ten of these cases will a doctor's visit be necessary. The result for the doctors in this practice, was that their work was perceived to be more enjoyable and meaningful and they spent longer with each patient. They also began to perform more procedures, such as electrocardiography. Moore and his colleagues (1973) have also provided evidence from their practice that a nurse can make decisions on a home visit which do not differ significantly, clinically or statistically, from those made by a doctor. However, most studies have been based on individual practices which may not be representative. Although the Report of the Joint Working Party on the Attachment of Nursing Services to General Practice (1970) supported first visits by nurses, more evaluative studies are needed before assessments can be made about their abilities.

Could either a further-trained nurse or a trained assistant also initially screen patients in the surgery and decide who needs to see the doctor? The British Medical Association (1977) have raised this possibility, only to reject it. It cannot be expected that general practitioners will willingly relinquish their role as the initial professional contact in the surgery until a clear definition of their role, beyond such basic descriptions, has been developed. Undoubtedly, nurses, with further training, could fulfil such a role. They have already shown that they are capable of exercising autonomy. For example, the Medicines Act Amendment Part 11 Order (1978) gives the industrial nurse a right to sign prescription-only medicines and to administer such medicines by injections, acting under a written instruction from a doctor. Hospital nurses also learn to discriminate between degrees of urgency in their observations of patients. There are many examples of nurses exercising autonomy and making diagnostic decisions. However, even if the nursing profession did decide that they would like to undertake this role, there is little likelihood of its successful development without the co-operation of the medical profession. But are nurses the best professionals to undertake a clinical and/or diagnostic role in the surgery?

6

A NURSE PRACTITIONER OR PHYSICIAN'S ASSISTANT: TO WHOM SHOULD THE DOCTOR DELEGATE?

If general practitioners are ever persuaded of the value of an extensive degree of delegation, should nurses be trained to a level similar to that of the nurse practitioner of the United States or Canada, or should new types of assistants be trained to undertake delegated tasks? Such an assistant could take over medical tasks currently performed by some nurses. The advantage of this would be that the nursing profession would then become more independent of the medical profession and lose one source of role conflict. The nurse would be free to concentrate on the essential task of nursing: nursing care. An analysis of this issue requires examination of the events leading to the development of the roles of the physician's assistant and nurse practitioner in the United States and Canada, as well as the current structure of these roles.

An assistant to the physician

There is no precise definition of the role of the physician's assistant. The appropriate role of such a person in a third-world country may be quite different from that required in an industrialized nation. Consequently, a number of different types of physician's assistant have emerged and a number of different labels describing such personnel have been introduced.

Despite the diversity in types and descriptions of such assistants, two levels of training and skill can be distinguished. The first level is that of personnel with eight or nine years of general education and a two- or three-year course of specialized training. Such personnel work under the supervision of doctors, and may provide the only daily contact with medical aid for many populations in rural areas of the world. For example, they are to be found in the Central African Republic, Guatemala, Iran, Kenya, the Republic of Vietnam, the Sudan, and the United Republic of Tanzania. Duke University in the United States has also instituted a course to train such personnel and other United States universities have followed their initiative. These health workers may be trained in diagnostic and treatment techniques, or only in the latter.

The second level of such personnel involves individuals with a limited amount of secondary education who, after a short training period, can perform simple medical and first-aid procedures. These workers are generally attached to village health posts serving a population of a few thousand. The prototypes of these workers are the barefoot doctors of the People's Republic of China.

It is the first type of health worker with which this section is concerned. This type of assistant has been described by the World Health Organisation (1975) as a health worker whose duties include diagnosis and treatment of minor illness. They are described as being auxiliaries to the physician and as under his, or her, supervision. This is the model which would be simulated if such personnel were ever introduced in Britain.

The interest in training physicians' assistants in the United States was primarily stimulated by academics and government officials who were concerned about the alleged shortage of general practitioners. General practice has long been held in low esteem in the United States and its prestige rating had inevitable repercussions on recruitment. The number of doctors in general practice fell from 76 per cent of all physicians in 1940 to 36 per cent in 1965 (Bonnet 1972). The interest in creating a new body of health practitioners to assist the physician, in order to increase the quantity of care dispensed, received further stimulus from efforts to utilize the skills of military medical corpsmen returning to civilian life at the end of the Vietnam war. The first physician's assistant training programme was subsequently inaugurated at Duke University in 1965. Estes (1969) has pointed out that the tasks physicians actually perform can be divided into those requiring the complex judgement that their education prepared them for, and those that require technical skills which may be learned through repetition. It is these latter skills that the physician's assistant is trained to perform at Duke University. One aim of the programme is to prepare the physician's assistant to do anything which the doctor can train him or her to do. Dr Eugene Stead, who was responsible for establishing the physician's assistant programme at Duke, suggested that assistants could eventually collect data from the patient, feed it into an automated clinical-decision system, and give the results to the physician (Stead 1968). However, their current role at Duke is basically technical, including the performance of such tasks as venepuncture, intubations of the gastrointestinal tract, intravenous infusions, the operation of instruments such as the electrocardiograph and respirator, the giving of medications, and keeping of progress records. This role is distinct from those relating to other programmes which confine their skills within a single specialty or to the performance of a specific technical procedure.

The programme at Duke is basically a twenty-four-month curriculum divided into a nine-month didactic period and a fifteen-month clinical portion. The admission requirements are a high-school diploma, or its equivalent, with courses in chemistry, algebra, and biology, and experience in the health field, for example as a corpsman or licensed practical nurse. Originally intended to provide the general practitioner and general internist with an assistant, the programme has developed and now provides assistants for all types of specialties.

Since the inception of the Duke programme, a considerable number of additional programmes have developed throughout the United States. The Medex programme, for example, was initiated by Dr Richard Smith in 1969 at the University of Washington, in collaboration with the State Medical Society. This programme recruits former medical corpsmen and nurses. Medex training provides three months of didactic study, followed by a twelve- to fifteen-month preceptorship under a physician willing to employ the Medex after training. Because of its success, this programme has also been replicated in other universities. In supervised remote practices, Medex alone can cope with ninety per cent of the patient contacts in an out-patient clinic. This is possible because Medex can perform many of the routine repetitive tasks which were previously performed by the physician but which do not require a physician's sophisticated level of training. Medex are also taught to act as the initial point of contact for patients and to decide which patients require referral to the doctor and which can be treated by the Medex alone. Protocols, or clinical flow charts, have been developed to assist the latter in clinical decision-making. These direct the Medex in determining what data to collect, and whether or not the patient needs to see the doctor. From experience gained using such algorithms at Dartmouth College in the United States, it has been established that they can be used safely and effectively (Tompkins and Johnson 1976).

Unfortunately, however, because of the terminological confusion surrounding assistants to the physician, no estimate of the numbers of such assistants can be made. All that is known is that by 1974 forty-eight training programmes had been accredited by the American Medical Association (Sadler, Sadler, and Bliss 1974).

A nurse practitioner

Dolan (1969) has argued that nurses, with further training, are a more logical choice as an assistant to the physician. Not only may nurses have the ability and knowledge to expand their roles in diagnostic and therapeutic areas, but they also have experience in acting as the doctor's assistant in addition to performing their own nursing functions. It is certainly true that it may be preferable to define the roles of existing health care professionals, and to consider their more effective organization, before introducing new types of personnel. Furthermore, in the United States and in Britain, nurses form the largest available pool of health manpower. There are currently large numbers of inactive registered nurses, some of whom have left their profession because of what they perceived to be the limited and unchallenging nature of conventional nursing roles (MacGuire 1969; Annandale Steiner 1979; Redfern 1979). However, the debate over whether nurses should expand their role to become assistants to the physician continues, even in the United States, where nurse practitioner programmes are established. The main reason that the issue has not been resolved within the nursing profession is that nursing itself has still not defined its own role and made explicit what is distinctive about it.

One of the reasons for the initial postponement of the nurse practitioner programme in the United States was this dilemma within nursing. Nursing leaders were approached by the American Medical Association in 1969 and invited to consider expanding the role of the nurse into that of a physician's assistant. It was proposed by Dr Eugene Stead, then the Chairman of the Department of Medicine at Duke University, and Thelma Ingles, who was on the faculty of the school of nursing, that graduates of the Duke School of Nursing would be trained to assume greatly expanded duties, working as assistants to physicians. This was to be a programme at master's degree level. After one year the programme was condemned by the National League of Nursing and was discontinued. It was during this period that the faculty of the Department of Medicine at Duke began to recruit discharged military corpsmen to perform duties in the cardiac catheterization laboratory, renal dialysis laboratory, and other similar areas. This was regarded as successful, and led to further consideration of the effective utilization of returning military medical corpsmen. Stead, aware of these developments, developed the concept of a training programme to equip the corpsmen to function as physicians' assistants. The internal politics of the situation were more complex than this brief description suggests. In 1970 the American Medical Association urged an expansion of the role of the nurse so that nurses could assist physicians (*American Medical Association News* 1970). However, Dorothy Cornelius (1970), the President of the American Nursing Association, argued that it was not the prerogative of one profession to speak for another and stated that such action would increase the shortage of nurses. Thus, Bonnet (1972) has suggested that the similar rejection of the Duke programme for nurse practitioners in the 1960s was because nurses felt such a suggestion was professionally compromising.

Consequently, the proposed expansion of the role of the nurse was temporarily postponed. Soon after the inauguration of the physician's assistant programmes many nurses began to feel that they should be undertaking this new role. Simultaneous developments occurred in Canada during this period. For example, after the development of the role of physician's assistant, the Canadian Nurses' Association (1970) argued that nurses constituted a large, readily available source of manpower who, with a little further training, could undertake greater medical responsibilities.

Nevertheless, the nursing profession appeared to perceive an element of professional threat in the introduction of new categories of health personnel. This may have been partly because physicians' assistants were also trained to perform technical procedures sometimes performed by nurses. Although nurses were reluctant to perform delegated medical duties because of a fear of losing their professional identity, they were equally reluctant to see their position usurped. Changes in professional duties may not only have role implications, but they may also have long-term effects on professional status and on relationships between different types of professionals. It is such long-term effects which are likely to be felt as threatening.

As a result of such feelings of threat among the nursing profession, nurse practitioner programmes began to emerge both in the United States and Canada. If the nursing profession had accepted Stead's initial effort to expand their role there may never have been a physician's assistant programme. Ironically, had there not been a physician's assistant programme, there may not have been a nurse practitioner programme. Thus, the nursing profession's concern with status brought into existence a rival group of health workers who seriously challenged their role.

There is less information available about nurse practitioners and their training than about physicians' assistants. Sadler, Sadler, and Bliss (1974) give details of approximately 128 programmes listed by the American Nursing Association in 1974. Of these, over half led to certification and the remainder led to a master's degree. All the programmes required entrants to be at least registered nurses. Programmes for master's degrees usually required a bachelor's degree in nursing. The different programmes varied in length from ten weeks to two years. Reedy (1978) has pointed out that programmes at Johns Hopkins consist of a four-month period of didactic instruction with concurrent clinical experience. This is followed by an eight-month period in the setting of the nurse's future employment. All the teaching is carried out by either a nurse practitioner or a physician.

Nurse practitioners are taught to take a complete medical history and to perform a physical examination. The curriculum for nurse practitioners referred to by Spitzer and Kergin (1973) includes interviewing and history taking, physical examination, prenatal and postnatal care, well-child assessment, evaluation and management of common acute and chronic disorders, and of common emotional and social disorders, geriatrics and the utilisation of community health and welfare services.

The distinction between a physician's assistant and a nurse practitioner

So what is the difference between these two types of personnel? A survey by the United States Departments of Health, Education and Welfare (1977) of the selection of both types of practitioner reveals that the physician's assistant places more emphasis on basic sciences compared with nurse practitioner programmes. It was felt by selectors that nurses would have experienced similar basic courses prior to entry to the nurse practitioner training programme. Physician's assistant programmes include surgery and emergency care skills in their training, in contrast again to nurse practitioner programmes. Nurses are expected to have previously acquired such skills. Consequently, nurse practitioner programmes are much shorter. But what are the distinctions between these two groups in practice, once they have been trained? Reedy (1978) has pointed out that one of the main distinctions between these types of practitioner is the stress on health. For example, physicians' assistants are oriented towards a disease model of their function, while nurse practitioners are oriented towards a model of health maintenance, or prevention. Reedy (1979) further points out that nurse practitioners have more autonomy than physicians' assistants as they are usually employed by institutions rather than by physicians. As a result, they tend to have a more equal relationship with doctors.

Because of a fear of losing their independent professional identity through adoption of an expanded medical role, nursing organizations frequently stress the distinctions between a physician's assistant and a nurse practitioner. The American Nurses' Association (1971), for example, has argued that calling a nurse practitioner a physician's assistant would have a detrimental effect on the individuality of nursing as distinct from medicine. It would also have a detrimental effect on the attempts of nursing to become an autonomous profession. As one of the commonly cited criteria for professional status is autonomy of action, the label of assistant to the physician would be a retrograde step in the nurses' fight for professional status. Thus, nursing organizations in the United States and Canada have stipulated that the nurse practitioner must be seen as an associate of the physician, rather than as an assistant.

However, the functions of the nurse practitioner still appear similar, in practice, to those of the various types of physician's assistant. The nurse practitioner may take medical histories, complete physical examinations, request and interpret laboratory tests and practise preventive medicine. Equally, the nurse practitioner may concentrate on performing a general range of technical procedures, on diagnostic and screening functions, or concentrate on more complex diagnostic or technical skills in a particular specialty. Where state laws permit, they may also prescribe drugs. As with the physician's assistant, many descriptive studies of the work of the nurse practitioner exist (Hadley 1976). The similarity of functions between the two groups leads one to ask whether similar roles are merely given different titles to satisfy the political interests of the nursing profession? This criticism would be valid only if nurses did not contribute to this role in a unique way. According to the previously mentioned nursing organizations, nursing practitioners do not simply offer a more health-conscious approach, but also contribute through their caring attitudes. It is this element of the nurse's work which nursing leaders like to believe is unique. More studies are undoubtedly needed comparing these two roles before any conclusions about the unique contribution made by the nurse practitioner can be drawn. In any case, the role of physician's assistant, nurse practitioner, and that of the physician will inevitably overlap.

A nurse practitioner or physician's assistant in Britain?

Role changes within one professional group may lead to changes in the roles of related professional groups. Such changes may also lead to different patterns of interaction between these groups and may even have long-term effects on their professional status. Any attempt, then, to change the role of one group may have implications for other groups working in the same area. Consequently, conflict between groups may be inevitable when attempts are made to change established patterns of work. The existence of potential conflict has implications for the type of personnel doctors may be willing to delegate to, and for the type of personnel willing to take on a technical and/or diagnostic role in the surgery. It also has implications for the willingness of doctors to delegate at all.

What are the advantages of nurses undertaking an expanded medical role in general practice and to what extent can potential conflict be minimized? Traditionally, nurses have been the main source of assistance to doctors. Many doctors may consequently feel reluctant to accept assistance from a new source. Reedy (1978) believes that, in Britain, only the nurse practitioner could survive, as the medical and nursing professions would both feel more threatened by the introduction of new types of health workers and use considerable power to oppose their introduction. A nurse practitioner may pose less of a threat to the medical profession than a specially trained physician's assistant, who could be perceived as an aspiring physician. It is possible that such a person may simply aim to undertake as many tasks within the role of the physician as possible. There is no evidence to support this fear. On the other hand, physicians may perceive nurses to be a greater threat as they are currently attempting to organize themselves as a profession. In contrast, the physician's assistant cannot aspire to professional status, as this implies the possession of an independent body of knowledge and there is little likelihood of assistants possessing such knowledge. However, doctors in Britain would probably find it difficult to accept working with new types of personnel in view of their traditional reluctance to introduce organizational innovations on a wide scale.

A nurse practitioner may also be more acceptable to the nursing profession in this country. Physicians' assistants in the United States and Canada perform many of the procedures undertaken by nurses as well as by doctors. It was this role overlap which led to conflict and to the eventual creation of a nurse practitioner role. On the other hand, nurses may be understandably reluctant to accept such a role unless it offered them a substantial degree of autonomy. Reedy (1978) has argued, for example, that British nurses are less subordinate in their relationships with doctors than are American nurses. This, he feels, partly explains why the role of the nurse practitioner has evolved in America but not in Britain.

Nurses are, in addition, a ready source of manpower as many are currently unemployed. It is possible that these nurses may find an expanded medical role in general practice attractive. If they would not have returned to nursing in its other forms, then the encouragement of such a role does not diminish the available source of nursing manpower. In fact, only one-quarter to one-third of nurses on the Register and the Roll of the General Nursing Council are actually practising. Of the remainder, 10 per cent are known to be over retirement age, and an unknown number may be dead. It has been estimated that there is a reserve of approximately 60 per cent of all qualified nurses who are not practising (Weightman 1978). Such wastage rates may often be due to nurses, who are predominantly female, interrupting their careers to raise children. Evidence that these individuals may find the role of the nurse practitioner attractive is provided by the findings of Reedy and his colleagues (1980b), which show that nurses working in surgeries work shorter hours than community nurses. The flexible hours of the former type of employment, and possibly of the nurse practitioner role, may be more popular among nurses with young families. Furthermore, the Dan Mason Nursing Research Committee (1967) confirmed this supposition in its survey of the attitudes and occupations of 6000 nurses. Those who were unemployed felt a choice of working hours and flexibility would induce them to return to nursing. These conditions were perceived as more important than salary because of their family commitments.

It could be argued that there is no need to employ more nurses to work in general practices to undertake delegated medical tasks, as such functions could be undertaken by nurses currently working in the community if they were given further training. Attached nurses are sometimes likely to be used as substitutes for employed nurses or treatment room nurses. However, the extent to which attached community nurses can be substituted for employed nurses in the treatment room is limited as the nature of the work of both types of nurse differs in a number of ways (Reedy *et al.* 1980b).

Hockey (1968) also found that few district nurses in her sample felt that they could have coped with additional work and over half believed that their present workload was too heavy. The Royal College of Nursing (1977) has argued that state registered nurses currently undertake work which could be performed by a state enrolled nurse. If this is the case, perhaps if these nurses working in the community delegated more of their work to state enrolled nurses and to nursing auxiliaries they would have more time to undertake delegated medical tasks. But would community or district nurses want to spend more time on medical functions? Treatment room work and community nursing are two distinct branches of nursing. It cannot be assumed that nurses who elected to work in the community, in a more caring type of role, would wish to spend more time in the surgery in a more technical role. They may not even wish to develop their diagnostic or assessment skills by performing initial home visits in the place of a doctor. However, Reedy and his colleagues (1980b) did find that many district nurses felt that in the future they would combine their work in patients' homes with work in general practitioners' surgeries. Moreover, many of them saw this as a worthwhile development. On the other hand, it is not known whether they would want to expand their roles in the surgery as extensively as nurse practitioners.

In the United States, several other arguments have been presented in favour of the creation of nurse practitioner posts, rather than physician's assistant posts. For example, the future career potential in the United States of physicians' assistants is still unknown, although it has been suggested (Conant 1974) that they are basically non-competitive and do not want sole responsibility. It is not known whether physicians' assistants will remain satisfied with their careers. In Russia feldshers may, after further study, become fully qualified doctors. However, many do not take advantage of this opportunity because they do not want further responsibility. According to Breytspraak and Pondy (1969) all that is known is that physicians' assistants find their own lack of identity to be a serious problem. This feeling is apparently mainly due to the proliferation of different types of assistant who have no unifying factor. But does the nurse practitioner experience less uncertainty? They may retain a sense of identity with the nursing profession, but only in so far as they practise their role within the context of providing nursing care. On the other hand, Storms (1973) has suggested that these nurses risk being ostracized by other nurses because they are supervised by members of another profession whilst performing the tasks of that profession: medicine.

Perhaps the main argument in favour of introducing nurse practitioners, rather than new types of personnel, is that nurses already possess a basic knowledge of medical science and would merely require an extension course to prepare them for an expanded role. Since in Britain we have no ready supply of returning medical corpsmen, as did the United States, we have no potential supply of physicians' assistants. It is possible that rejected medical school applicants might undertake this role. Such applicants, however, are likely to feel frustrated as physicians' assistants if medicine was their first career choice.

On the other hand, Fendall (1972) has argued that expanded medical roles for nurses are a waste of the nurse's previous training, divert the nurse from his or her chosen vocation, and are not in the best interests of nursing as a profession. To divert a nurse to medical care is thus seen as illogical, especially when such personnel are often themselves in short supply. However, the high rate of nurse wastage has already been emphasized. While little research has been done on this issue in Britain, research in the United States suggests that high wastage rates are due to lack of direct patient care by nurses who, upon promotion, are forced to undertake managerial functions (Sadler, Sadler, and Bliss 1974). It is possible that the performance of medical tasks might enhance nurses' satisfaction with their work as such a role would involve them in direct contact with patients. It may also increase their self-esteem as they would be performing procedures requiring a higher degree of technical skill. Unfortunately, the effect of the development of the nurse practitioner role on the status of the nursing profession and on the level of nurses' work satisfaction has been neglected by social scientists.

Undeniably, to assume that nurses could readily undertake a role which would infringe upon that of the medical profession does reveal some misunderstanding of the role of the nurse. Before the advent of scientific medicine the nurse was the principal worker in the hospital. With scientific advance, physicians and surgeons became the dominant figures in these institutions and the nurse became a mere cog in the medical machine. Although doctors began to rely on nurses for assistance, nurses already had their own set of tasks which were not inherited from the doctor: those relating to caring for patients rather than diagnosing or curing them. Consequently, the role of the nurse today is ambiguous in that it is a mixture of medical tasks and nursing care. The nursing profession maintains that nursing care is the essential feature of their role, although this has yet to be satisfactorily defined. Nurses may thus regard the role of the nurse practitioner as taking them further away from caring and from a satisfactory role definition. From this point of view, the introduction of new types of health personnel to perform delegated medical tasks may free nurses to concentrate on the caring aspect of their role. However, as was previously pointed out, the introduction of physicians' assistants would affect the role of the nurse, and nurses are likely to feel threatened as a result (Bowling 1980e).

Nevertheless the extent to which nurses in Britain already perform some of the tasks performed by physicians' assistants and nurse practitioners abroad makes them the most likely personnel to undertake an expanded medical role. As MacGuire (1980) has argued, nurses should not be misled into thinking that in adopting a nurse practitioner role they would be introducing anything new. They would simply be cultivating and expanding what already existed. As long as this was done within the context of nursing care, then it is not necessarily to the detriment of nursing as a profession. With increasing debate on the issue of delegation it is possible that at some stage in the future we will be faced with the problem of systematizing or rejecting an expanded nurse role in general practice. If such a role is rejected for nurses, then a debate on whether to introduce physicians' assistants may emerge. Whatever course of action is taken partly depends on how nursing decides to define its role. Whether a nurse practitioner or physician's assistant is introduced, role changes within nursing and general practice are inevitable. For this reason, the main sources of opposition to such schemes are likely to be the nursing and medical professions themselves. The role and status insecurity experienced by general practitioners throughout their history has been documented. In order to more fully understand the likely opposition of nurses to such organizational changes a brief description of nursing history is necessary.

7

PROFESSION OF NURSING: THE PROBLEM OF STATUS AND IMPLICATIONS FOR ROLE EXPANSION

Little research has been undertaken with the aim of documenting the attitudes of nurses and their professional bodies towards the performance of delegated medical duties, either by themselves or by other health practitioners. However, nursing organizations in Britain have indicated that they perceive overlapping medical and nursing roles to be outside the professional interests of nursing. For example, the Briggs Report emphasized the distinctions between the caring role of the nurse and the diagnostic and therapeutic role of the doctor (Report of the Committee on Nursing 1972). The Report stated that only when the unique role of the nurse has been clearly defined will it be possible to examine areas of overlap between the role of the nurse and that of the doctor. The reasoning underlying this attitude is interlinked with the role ambiguity suffered by nursing today, and the consequent feeling of role threat. Current attempts to define the unique role of the nurse are in turn interlinked with the struggle of nursing to establish itself as a profession equal to medicine. It is this struggle which influences the responses of nursing leaders towards the issue of intermediate level health practitioners. The Briggs Report, for example, explicitly stated its disapproval of the nurse becoming a medical assistant on the grounds that this could jeopardize the caring functions of the nurse. The profession is currently emphasizing these caring functions in an attempt to establish professional individuality. Both the Briggs Report and the Joint Report of the Royal College of Nursing and the Royal College of General Practitioners (1974) indicated that nurses should not undertake medical tasks simply because doctors find them time consuming or trivial, on the grounds that this would be a misuse of nursing skills. The Royal College of Nursing (1979) has recently revealed a greater willingness to thoroughly discuss the issue of an expanded role for the nurse in this area. The College now believes that such an expanded role may be envisaged, on condition that performing delegated medical tasks is never considered to be the most important function of the nurse. However, they have not issued any guidelines nor listed any tasks considered suitable for delegation. In fact, they rejected the suggestion that they should do so. Nor have they offered any type of definition of an expanded nursing role.

On the whole, it appears that until the nursing profession has successfully defined its role in a way which will establish its independent identity, the fear of being consumed by the medical profession will remain. The implication is that until nursing has achieved a greater degree of professional status, for which an independent role definition is essential, then nurses are unlikely to view favourably any role changes within other professions which might affect them. To what extent has nursing achieved professional status?

Nursing as a profession

Whether a trait, functionalist, historical, Weberian, or any other perspective on the professions is adopted (see Johnson 1972), nursing cannot be regarded as a profession in the full meaning of the term. For example, in comparison with medicine, the training of the nurse is shorter, their body of knowledge is less specialized, academic affiliation with the universities has only recently been initiated, and nurses possess less autonomy from supervision or societal control than do the more established professions of medicine and law. Thus, although nurses are typically referred to as professionals, they do not enjoy privilege and autonomy to the same extent as doctors (Bowling 1980b).

The position of nursing in the nineteenth century

Since the mid-nineteenth century nurses have been struggling to enhance their professional status. The history of nursing certainly dates from the Middle Ages, when nursing was undertaken by nuns who were both educated and devoted. When Henry VIII dissolved the monasteries in 1539, however, these religious orders were dispersed. Hospitals then became charity institutions and the newly emerging type of nurse was illiterate and certainly not dedicated. During the early part of the nineteenth century the nurse was simply an untrained attendant. By the 1920s, however, a General Nursing

Council had been established which regulated nurse training and nursing schools within hospitals, and which conducted the examinations by which admission to the State Register was gained. This process of rapid change was effected through several mediums. Medical advances meant that doctors needed assistants to perform routine tasks. This development occurred at a time of demographic imbalance which created a large number of single middle-class women who made ideal recruits to nursing. The emancipation of women and their consequent demand for employment also affected the development of nursing as a suitable and respectable form of employment. The process of reform within this occupation initiated by Florence Nightingale and Mrs Bedford Fenwick was successful only because the social situation favoured change.

Conflicts soon arose between these two pioneers of reform. Mrs Bedford Fenwick was the leader of the movement which aimed to increase the professional status of nursing by introducing a system of licensure and lengthening the period of nurse training. Florence Nightingale strongly opposed this movement as she felt that nursing was simply a calling, the status of which was dependent primarily on the personal qualities of the nurse. How did these women affect the professional status of nursing?

Florence Nightingale became well known for her nursing efforts during the Crimean War. As a result of her work the public provided her with sufficient subscriptions to enable her to open a School of Nursing at St Thomas's Hospital. Abel Smith (1960) has described how the minimum of educational attainment but the maximum of moral stature were the essential requirements for entry into the school. Recruitment tended to be confined to those from lower middle-class backgrounds, such as the daughters of small farmers and well-educated domestic servants, and from the higher social classes. By such means the image of the nurse changed from that of an old hag to that of a dedicated lady. Nightingale established a hierarchical ordering of nurses, with matrons at the apex. Prior to her innovations, lay nurses had been under the authority of men (doctors) and the consequent treatment of nurses as servants had been a major obstacle to morale among nurses (Shyrock 1959). However, the adoption by Nightingale of an all-female organizational hierarchy within nursing meant that the female employees of the hospital, the nurses, became responsible to a matron for all but medical orders. Since doctors were preoccupied with clinical matters, and since lay administration was developed much later, the nursing hierarchy became the administrative structure of the English voluntary hospital.

It was this Nightingale system which eventually spread throughout Britain. However, this did not occur immediately. Throughout the nineteenth century the demand for nurses increased and as hospitals expanded the demand exceeded supply. In response to this situation, workhouse infirmaries and other local authority hospitals began their own training schemes, since, for the most part, Nightingale's students tended to confine their practice to the higher status, private institutions. Consequently, the quality of nurse training began to vary. At the same time, some hospitals began using student nurses as a form of cheap labour rather than preparing them for their careers. At this time, Dr and Mrs Bedford Fenwick became leaders in the movement to increase the status of nursing by introducing a system of licensure and lengthening the period of training for nurses. This campaign was strengthened by the new spirit of professionalism which was emerging in all occupations. Nurses also had before them an ideal example of the process of professionalism in the form of the medical profession.

Mrs Bedford Fenwick's most notable achievement was the state registration of nurses in 1887. In that year, the British Nurses' Association, of which she was founder, announced its desire to establish a General Registry of Nurses. Such a register had been provided by Parliament for physicians in the 1850s. As with the medical profession, the function of this register was not only to protect the public, but also to protect the profession from unqualified practitioners. Mrs Bedford Fenwick had demanded State registration, admission to the register after three years' nursing education followed by examination, the accreditation of nursing schools, the elimination of salaries for student nurses, and the creation of organizations under nurses' control by which they could administer registration, accreditation and other professional affairs. Florence Nightingale fought such proposals, on the grounds that national registration would include the worst as well as the best nurses since it could certify nothing about a nurse's character. To Nightingale, character was all-important. The outcome of several years' controversy was that the British Nurses' Association was granted a Royal Charter in 1893 and was permitted to maintain a list of those nurses who desired to be included. However, it was given no exclusive right to register nurses, nor any control over nursing education. The fight for greater professional status was only partly won. In 1916 a new force in favour of registration emerged in the form of the College of Nursing Limited. However, it was not until 1928 that the College was given a Royal Charter. Its principal aims were: to promote the education and training of nurses and the advancement of nursing as a profession, to promote uniformity of curriculum, to recognize approved nursing schools, to make and maintain a register of people to whom certificates of proficiency or of training and proficiency had been granted, and to promote legislation in Parliament which was in the interests of nursing, in particular statutes related to nursing education, organization, protection, and State recognition.

The process of professionalization after 1916

The first task to which the College of Nursing addressed itself was State registration. Registration, in principle, was approved by the Select Committee on Registration of 1904–5. Each year, from 1904 to 1914, a Registration Bill was placed before Parliament and each year it was rejected. It was not until 1919 that registration became law. Just as the year 1858 saw the partial establishment of functional autonomy within the medical profession, so the year 1919 saw its partial establishment within nursing. The creation of a system of registration and licensing led to the essential first steps which enabled nursing to control the recruitment and training of its members. However, this control was not as complete as that achieved by the medical profession. The 1919 Act created the General Nursing Council which was the statutory body responsible for nurse examinations, syllabuses, disciplinary procedures, and approval of training schools, as well as the maintenance of a register of nurses. However, its autonomy was limited as the decisions and recommendations of the Council were subject to the approval of the Minister of Health. Rules concerning admission to the register were to be operated only with the approval of this minister. Every rule was to be passed by the House of Commons and House of Lords. Furthermore, a nurse did not even chair the General Nursing Council itself for six years. The first chairperson was a former barrister. Even today, doctors still sit on this Council, although no nurses sit on the General Medical Council.

In addition, the criteria necessary for a good nursing training were omitted from the Bill, to be disputed by the Council. As the Council was heterogeneous in composition, its members represented many different sections in nursing; debates continued over whether and under what conditions existing nurses should be admitted to the register, the training and examination requirements for registered nurses, and the criteria for granting approval to nurse training schools. Moreover, the 1919 Act did not generate uniformity of practice as had been hoped. Although State examinations were held from 1925, the General Nursing Council did not regulate the training syllabus, nor did it possess more powers to inspect and approve schools. As a result the quality of training remained variable.

The autonomy of the nursing profession was also threatened by the Government. Politicians felt that exclusiveness would exacerbate the alleged shortage of nursing staff. Thus, the plans by the General Nursing Council to make training a necessary condition for admission to the register and to impose stringent educational tests on new entrants were overruled by Parliament. Furthermore, the administrative body responsible for registering nurses and approving nursing schools was dominated by matrons, who were responsive to the staffing needs of hospitals. As a consequence, service demands were given priority over professional criteria. In addition many hospitals were permitted to have nursing schools and thus apprenticeship training remained.

The next event to affect the structure of nursing was the 1943 Nurses' Bill which introduced a lower grade of nurse, the state enrolled nurse. The continuing shortage of nurses had led to the gradual realization that not all nursing duties could be performed by one grade of nurse. The introduction of a second grade of nurse who would undertake a course with an emphasis on practical work was thus proposed. This suggestion was accepted by the nursing profession only after legislation restricting the title of nurse to these two grades was agreed. These recommendations were subsequently implemented in the 1943 Nurses' Bill. The existence of two grades of nurse, and the utilization of untrained nursing auxiliaries, is responsible for much of the role confusion in nursing today. Lower grade nurses perform many of the basic caring tasks, for example the bathing of patients, which a number of nurses regard as within the proper (caring) role of the higher grade nurse.

The National Health Service Act of 1946 next brought nurses, along with the medical profession as a whole, directly into Government employment. As with doctors, this Act implied State recognition of the monopoly of trained nurses who were either registered or enrolled by the General Nursing Council. To some extent, it went part of the way towards establishing public belief in the occupation's competence, knowledge and skill – necessary criteria for autonomy.

The current status of nursing as a profession

The State employment of nurses has had more serious implications for the development of nursing as a profession. The Government has had no interest in maintaining the professional interests of nursing, unless this were to result in an enhanced level of recruitment. For example, the General Nursing Council currently wishes to raise the educational qualifications for trainees for the register from two 'O' level GCE passes. This request has been refused by the Department of Health and Social Security. Of course, the recommendations of the General Nursing Council have been subject to the approval of the Minister of Health since the 1919 Act. State employment merely seemed to reinforce this external control. In such circumstances, it is difficult to see how nursing can improve its knowledge base in order to enable its members to possess the same professional status as the classical professions with their university-based training.

What criteria of professional status does nursing either satisfy or fail to satisfy? One necessary criterion for such status is generally held to be a disciplined educational process resulting in formal recognition. Nursing does possess this, but nurse training is not extensive, especially in comparison with that of doctors. The training of a state registered nurse takes three years, and that of an enrolled nurse two years. In contrast, the training of a doctor takes five years onwards. Moreover, most nurses are trained in hospital nursing schools, largely on an apprenticeship basis, with unsystematic exposure to theoretical and tested knowledge. Such programmes cannot provide a sufficient grounding to enable nurses to acquire a body of theory and knowledge necessary for professional status. Although a limited amount of university training is available for nurses, there appears to be no strong emphasis on advanced education. Few practising nurses hold degrees and many nurses hold unfavourable attitudes towards degrees in nursing. It is generally believed that academic study does not equip nurses with necessary practical skills (House 1977). Thus British nurses appear to feel that nursing requires dedication rather than education and the influence of Florence Nightingale remains. Reinkemeyer (1966) has suggested that nursing in Britain can become an academic subject only if the glorification of practical nursing is abandoned and the quality of teaching, learning, theory construction, and the formulation of a body of knowledge through research are emphasized instead. This, in turn, will depend on nursing developing a stronger relationship with the universities.

The situation in Britain contrasts strongly with that in the United States where, as early as 1965, the American Nurses' Association publicly stated that nurse training programmes should be located within the universities. By 1972 less than half the nurse training schemes in the United States were associated with hospitals. The majority of nurse graduates in that year held degrees. In contrast, in Britain in 1972 there were a total of eleven experimental schemes for university nursing programmes and less than half of one per cent of nurses graduating in that year held a degree or diploma in addition to the registration requirements. Even today few nurses hold degrees (Facts About Nursing 1972–73; Davies 1978). Unsurprisingly, in 1972 the Report of the Committee on Nursing (Briggs) commented on the low level of recruitment into nursing of candidates with 'A' level GCE passes. Only 1654 of the 14 195 entrants into nurse training in 1970 to 1971 had one or more 'A' level passes. As high-grade 'A' level passes are often the norm for medical students, the differences between medical and nursing graduates in terms of educational status are wide.

The Government still refuses to implement legislative changes relating to the educational status of nurses, so educational differences will remain. Even the recommendations of the Committee on Nursing Education which reported in 1964 (Platt Report) were rejected. Admittedly the Nurses, Midwives and Health Visitors Act (1979) has been passed, arising out of the recommendations of the Briggs Committee, and consequently in 1980 four national boards were set up, representing England, Scotland, Wales, and Northern Ireland. The function of these boards is to oversee training and to be responsible for discipline. In addition, the statutory nursing bodies have been replaced by the Central Nursing, Midwifery and Health Visiting Council for the United Kingdom. Thus the Act has dissolved a number of nursing bodies, including the General Nursing Council. The new Central Council has as its principal aim the improvement of standards of training and professional conduct for nurses, midwives, and health visitors. In the future it will be responsible for preparing and maintaining a register of these professional groups. It will decide what evidence of qualifications is needed for registration, what fees to charge, and other professional details. The Council will draw up rules for the removal of nurses from the register in situations of misconduct and will set up disciplinary committees to cover these matters.

The most significant aspect of the 1979 Act from the point of view of the professionalization of nursing is that the system of nurse training will be changed. However, these changes were not delineated in the legislation but were left to the new bodies to determine. The Briggs Committee suggested that there should be a compulsory basic nursing qualification before commencement of registration courses. In effect, this would mean the abolition of the present system of training for state enrolled nurses and state registered nurses; and instead all nurses would study for some basic qualification. Briggs also envisaged the separation of nursing schools from hospitals and suggested that 200 to 300 colleges of nursing should be set up. Whether these changes will occur remains to be seen, but if this were the case the status of nursing would be enhanced, especially if student nurses were no longer treated as apprentices.

The lack of adequate training and education has led to a situation in which nurses fail to satisfy the criteria of professionalism in a further sense. Nursing does not possess a unique theoretical body of knowledge since its knowledge base is still drawn largely from experience. Thus, the special area of nurses' competence is less well defined in comparison with that of medicine. One of the most persistent problems faced by nursing is that of defining what nursing is and what is distinctive about it. The lack of agreement over the role definition of the nurse can only weaken attempts to enhance the functional autonomy of nurses. The problem stems partly from the close historical relationship between medicine and nursing. Both are used in the clinical care of the patient. As a result of this role overlap, nurses are seeking to identify their unique contribution to care in an administrative field. Thus nursing in Britain is increasingly focused around management or administration, rather than techniques of patient care. Nursing has adopted this role in an attempt to escape the subordination they have experienced in relationship to the medical profession, as well as to attempt to locate an area of work over which it can claim and maintain a monopoly. The recommendations of the Report of the Committee on Senior Nursing Staff Structure of 1966 (Salmon Report) reinforced this trend with its emphasis on nursing hierarchies and management functions.

Until the late-1900s, the function of nurses was to care for patients. They performed duties such as the washing and dressing of patients and even the laundering of bandages. However, once medical practitioners established themselves in hospital settings nurses increasingly performed delegated medical duties. They became assistants to doctors as well as performing their own caring tasks. With the development of medical technology, the caring and curing processes began to overlap and nurses increasingly became the servants of doctors. The medical profession became dominant. Consequently nursing came to be regarded as a paramedical occupation. As Freidson has pointed out in the *International Encyclopedia of Social Science*, the very term paramedical implies a degree of subordination to medicine. The dominance of the medical profession means that all the work done by paramedical staff is subject to the order of the physician.

Thus because of this role overlap with the medical profession, attempts by nurses to define the unique clinical contribution of nursing to patient care have met with variable degrees of success. Apart from the emphasis on management skills, one direction taken has been the development of the role of the clinical nurse specialist. However, a unique body of knowledge has still not been developed. Has nursing any unique clinical skills around which a body of knowledge could be developed? Florence Nightingale held that nursing was not the unwanted residue of medicine and that the only similarity between these two professions is that they both revolve around sick people (Nightingale 1859). Hector (1973) has argued that the uniqueness of the nurse's role, in contrast to that of the doctor, is that the nurse is constantly with the patient, providing care and preparation for recovery. It could be argued that the caring function of the nurse is often performed by the relatives and friends of the patient, therefore, how can it be called unique? The Report of the Committee on Nursing (1972) counter-argued this point with the statement that patients and their families need additional help and that this help is often highly specialized and complex. Significantly, however, a recent study (Rosenthal *et al.* 1980) showed how nurses in one hospital typically delegated normal caring functions to patients' relatives to enable them to concentrate on their administrative role. In any case, this caring function is not based on a body of knowledge. Nursing practice is based upon experience rather than theory.

When attempting to persuade others of the unique role of the nurse, nurses rely on definitions with no scientific foundations. For example, one of the most quoted and respected definitions of nursing is that of Henderson, who argues that the unique function of the nurse is to assist the patient to perform activities leading to better health, or a peaceful death, that he or she would normally perform unaided, given the strength, will and knowledge (Henderson 1967). While many similar definitions exist, others have attempted to make more simplistic definitions between the medical and nursing professions. Fritz and Murphy (1966) have identified the roles of nursing as primarily caring–comforting, and secondarily curing. They argue that curing is the primary role of the physician and therefore the secondary role of the nurse. However, this caring role of the nurse, which is increasingly being emphasized, is usually delegated to nursing auxiliaries, if not families, while, as previously indicated, nurses themselves concentrate upon the managerial aspects of their work. Of course the current emphasis on the caring role of the nurse is partly a response of those nurses who resent the administrative role they are forced to undertake the higher up the status ladder they go.

The debate over the proper role of the nurse continues, and even the implementation of the nursing process in many hospitals has not helped to resolve it. This gives a more personal system of care, which includes an assessment of nursing needs and an evaluation of the nursing care given. Should nurses concentrate on bedside nursing or on managerialism? Does the future of nursing lie in these fields or in the direction of the clinical nurse specialist acting as a consultant in particular fields of care, for example stoma care? Such questions remain unanswered.

While attempting to define its role and to establish independent professional status, nursing is faced with the dilemma that its work is not simply controlled by nursing practitioners but by medical practitioners. The reorganization of nursing into a greater hierarchical management structure as a result of the Salmon Report was an attempt to make nurses responsible to other, more senior, nurses. However, the nurse still cannot ignore the orders of the physician. It is the physician who possesses ultimate responsibility for the patient. The lack of autonomy within nursing, and the lack of decision-making and collaborative skills possessed by nurses has recently been demonstrated (Rosenthal *et al.* 1980). These authors also provide much evidence of the continuing subservience of nurses to doctors and show that, despite the fact that nurses were critical of certain medical practices, they were unlikely to express criticism in the presence of a doctor. At present, autonomy of action in nursing is lacking where patient care is concerned.

Autonomy of action – or discretionary authority and judgement – is delegated by society to selected occupations on the assumption that this is in the public interest. Of course, as has been illustrated, in practice the situation is more complex than this, since political interests intervene. However, while nurses may at times possess this authority and judgement in practice, as for example in the case of Sisters who sometimes seem to control the running of accident and emergency departments, in principle they do not. Hughes, Hughes, and Deutscher's study (1958) found that doctors frequently fail to fully exercise their authority and judgement and that nurses may exercise more judgement than they are legally entitled to. However, the nurse's authority is still theoretically limited. Where the nurse is responsible for a respirator or drip, the doctor is still looked to for decisions. Nurses still carry out doctors' orders. Of course, not all doctors possess complete autonomy. Junior doctors are controlled by their senior colleagues, but they are not controlled by members of another profession, at least in the sphere of clinical decision making. It is difficult to see how nurses can enhance their degree of autonomy of action while the medical profession is so dominant. It has been argued that one of the problems of such a female-based profession is that women have traditionally tended to defer to men (Etzioni 1969). If this argument is valid, difficulties may be inevitable in the event of nursing attempting to enhance its professional autonomy of action and hence its status.

Lack of certainty about the nurse's role has led to further problems within nursing: role strain. For example, although the nurse's administrative function may lead to independence, it also poses a major dilemma in that it results in the divorce of senior nurses from clinical work. One of the main reasons for choosing nursing as an occupation is that it is seen as a practical way of helping people. The caring image of the nurse is so pervasive that there are constant exhortations being made, imploring nurses to return to their traditional bedside role. Role confusion and strain are inevitable in a profession which attracts women who see themselves as bedside nurses and who then find that promotion and salary increases depend on upward mobility through a hierarchical administrative route. Other studies found that when nurses discover they cannot always act in a manner consistent with their own self-image, they tend to hold more critical and dissatisfied attitudes towards their seniors (Malone 1961, 1964; Berkowitz and Malone 1968).

Popular images of nursing contrast with reality. Furthermore, while both popular and student nurse images of nursing emphasize the practical, caring nature of this occupation this very image also leads to perceptions of nursing as a low-status occupation. Doctors, for example, have put forward low-status images of the traditional type of nurse (Hughes, Hughes, and Deutscher 1958; Hector 1973). In contrast to medicine which enjoys high prestige, especially that which is hospital based (Cartwright and Anderson 1981), a survey by National Opinion Polls Limited, albeit in 1966, found that nearly 26 per cent of the public rated secretarial and teaching work higher than nursing in a scale of first choice of occupation. Although the prestige of nursing may increase in the future as it becomes university based, at present recruitment to nursing is inevitably affected by such images. They may not only lead to dissatisfactions within nursing, and be responsible for some wastage, but will also ultimately affect the professional status of nursing.

Definitional problems in nursing, and the lack of a knowledge base, are directly related to the lack of a research base in nursing. A body of knowledge can be developed only through research. Thus, to be granted the rewards of an established profession, such as autonomy and prestige, nursing will have to illustrate through research that its members command an esoteric knowledge base and skills which enable them to accomplish their task more efficiently and with better results than the layman. At present, research in nursing is a relatively new field of endeavour, despite earlier encouragement by the Reports of the Committee on Senior Nursing Staff Structure (1966) and the Working Party on Management Structure in the Local Authority Nursing Services (1969). Despite the creation of nursing research liaison officer posts at regional health authority level, the development of nursing research has been slow.

Lack of research in nursing is not merely due to lack of financial support. A major problem is the lack of highly qualified nurses capable of conducting a rigorous inquiry into the clinical practice of their profession. As has been previously pointed out, educational standards within nursing are low. Even in the United States, where all nurses are actively encouraged to undertake degree programmes, few nurses undertake or complete doctoral theses based on research training and original investigatory work (Lysaught 1974).

In terms of the many trait theories of professional status, nursing fails to satisfy the criteria of professionalism in other senses. For example, if a profession is characterized by the level of commitment among its members then the position of nursing is ambivalent. As Anderson (1968) has pointed out, the level of commitment among nurses is low in comparison with that among doctors. Since nursing is a predominantly female occupation, it has a high proportion of part-time members and members with a shorter working life. Manpower wastage and absentee rates are also high (MacGuire 1969; Mercer 1979). This is often due to childbearing and family rearing activities. Anderson (1968) has also argued that this is an unfavourable base on which to build a strong professional group, because any profession needs a high proportion of professionals from which to recruit for leadership, training, and other senior positions. This may explain why male nurses have occupied a disproportionate number of middle-tier administrative posts in nursing.

On the other hand, nursing does satisfy one important criterion of professional status. It possesses its own professional association which has a Royal Charter: the Royal College of Nursing. Only qualified nurses are admitted to the College, including those in training. Untrained nursing auxiliaries are excluded from membership although they comprise over a quarter of all nursing staff. This is one reason why the Confederation of Hospital Service Employees can claim a higher rate of nurse membership than the Royal College of Nursing. The College has approximately 29 000 trainee nurse members and 75 800 trained members. It is not possible to estimate what proportion of all trained nursing staff or those in training are members of the College. This is because the number of agency nurses and the number of nurses operating in the private sector is unknown. Moreover, the figures for nurses working in the National Health Service in Scotland and Northern Ireland are unavailable. The number of trained nurses working in the English National Health Service is 353 320, and the number of trainees is 74 894. In terms of these figures, membership of the College appears low. In terms of professional status, membership of professional associations may reflect the extent to which a professional culture exists. This culture may be defined as the organization, development and passing on of skills to new members. Nurse training schools perform this function. However, if membership of professional bodies is low then this culture may become fragmented.

The relationship between nurses and others is defined in a code of ethics which states normative requirements and emphasizes the professional's responsibilities towards the layman. In this respect nurses share a similar code of ethics to doctors. However, despite the fact that nursing does satisfy certain requirements of professional status, such as a Council responsible for restricting entry to the profession and maintaining standards and regulating training, in addition to other prerequisites such as a code of ethics, nursing still remains a semi-profession.

Of course, when the medical profession achieved a substantial degree of functional autonomy as early as 1858, such criteria had not been met. Unique historical factors at that time contributed to their success along with the fact that medical practitioners shared a social and class background with the ruling élite. This led to identification and a similarity of interests which further strengthened practitioners' demands for a recognized professional status. In contrast, nurses are rarely recruited from the professional classes. Moreover, whilst historical factors enabled nursing to create a more respectable image of itself, the current situation does not favour an increase in its professional status. For example, the interests of nursing as a profession, and the interests of the State in maintaining sufficient numbers of recruits to nursing, are in direct opposition. This conflict has inevitable repercussions on standards of nurse training and education, and consequently on role and status.

In view of the debate over the proper role of the nurse, and the attempts to define nursing's unique contribution to patient care, it is hardly surprising that little agreement exists among nurses themselves over which tasks are within the scope of their role and which belong to other professionals (Kurtz and Flaming 1963; Gilmore, Bruce, and Hunt 1974). This dilemma illustrates the consequences of an occupational group aspiring to professional status while overlooking or minimizing the intellectual or scientific base of professional service.

In recognition of their semi-professional status, nurses are beginning to resist the dominance of the medical profession and attempting to define their own unique role, thus moves to delegate more medical tasks to them may well be resisted. Even the introduction of new types of health practitioners to perform such tasks may be rejected in nursing's present state of role confusion. As in the United States, new practitioners are likely to be perceived as threatening and as increasing role ambiguity. Thus, nursing's fear of being consumed by medicine may lead to a position of rigid task demarcation, which is not necessarily in the interests of the health service or the consumer. Although throughout its history nursing has often altered the nature of its role in response to medical discoveries and the development of new specialties, the current emphasis on professionalism may hinder such changes in the future. Doctors may be as resistant as nurses to role change.

Because any attempt to alter the role of one occupational group usually has implications for other groups working in the same area, potential conflict inevitably exists between doctors and nurses over role definitions. The basic problem appears to be, given the desirability of an expanded nurse role from the point of view of efficiency, how to organize this role in order to minimize conflicts of interests and without having detrimental effects on the professional status of any one group.

8

THE INTERVIEWS WITH DOCTORS

Because so little is known about the delegation of medical tasks in general practice and about general practitioners' and primary care nurses' attitudes in this area, a small survey of these professionals was undertaken. The aim of the survey was to document their practices and views. Only when their attitudes have been more fully understood will it be possible to predict the extent to which delegation will become more widespread in the future.

The sample of general practitioners

The study was carried out in four urban areas of England and Wales: Kingston-on-Thames, Croydon, Swansea, and Newport. Although the areas themselves were selected, within each area a simple random sample of twenty general practitioners was taken from the lists of the local Family Practitioner Committees. Sixty-eight of the eighty doctors sampled were successfully interviewed after initial contact by telephone. This gave a response rate of 85 per cent. All the interviews were carried out by the author between April and August 1977. The doctors who responded reflected characteristics common to the total population of general practitioners, such as year of graduation, number of partners, proportion of females, proportion born outside the UK, and the proportion operating an appointment system. The doctors who responded did not differ significantly from those who did not in terms of these characteristics or in terms of qualifications possessed.

The study areas

A small number of concentrated urban areas was chosen for the study because the interviewing was carried out by the author alone.

Inevitably, the non-randomness of the selection of the study areas limits the general applicability of the data. However, there is little reason to believe that the results do not reflect the views and practices of many doctors and nurses working in primary care in urban settings.

As the following descriptions illustrate, the study areas were quite distinct from each other:

Kingston-on-Thames is an affluent London borough and the administrative centre of Surrey. It is a Royal Borough and is situated in pleasant surroundings in which the River Thames is a central feature. A thriving market town, its market is one of the oldest in the country, dating back to 1240. The area has not, however, escaped the development of modern industry and housing estates. It has a population of approximately 135 600.

Croydon is a fairly affluent but more mixed area than Kingston. Before its absorption into Greater London it was Surrey's largest town. It has a population of 330 660 which makes it the largest, in terms of population, of the London boroughs. It is also as large as, and in many cases larger than, many provincial cities. It has the largest number of homes and the largest young population within Greater London. Over the past twenty years it has experienced a vast increase in office accommodation, making Croydon one of the major centres of office growth in the whole country, outside inner London.

A far less affluent area than either Kingston or Croydon, Swansea was once the victim of the dereliction left by the decline of the heavy metal industry and is now the victim of economic decline and consequently has a high level of unemployment. The second largest city in Wales, after Cardiff, it is a centre where modern industries have been attempting to develop and in which the port has played an important part in its economy. However, Swansea itself is surrounded by wooded and grassed areas and is close to the Gower Peninsular, scheduled as an area of outstanding natural beauty. Situated in West Glamorgan, it is a university town and has a population of nearly 200 000.

Newport, a far poorer area, also with a high level of unemployment, is a centre of attempted industrial development and an important seaport. Situated in Gwent, on the borders of England and Wales, it combines a strange mixture of pastoral charm and the gloom of the South Wales coalfield, although the coalfields are at least five miles away. The borough has a population in excess of 136 000 and a further million people live within twenty miles of the borough.

These four contrasting areas reflect different cultures: the English and the Welsh. It was hoped that they would also reflect a variety of medical practice.

The interviews

The interviews usually took place in the doctors' surgeries, and most lasted between one and a half and two and a half hours. A semi-structured interviewing schedule was used, designed to produce both qualitative and quantitative insights into doctors' attitudes towards delegation. It was felt necessary to supplement closed questions with open-ended questions because the subject matter was complex and the relevant dimensions were largely unknown. Doctors' views were probed in depth whenever possible, although always in a non-directive way. Ample opportunity was allowed for free responses. On such a complex issue, this method was felt to provide a good indication of whether the respondent had any information about the subject, whether he or she had a clearly formulated opinion about it, and how strongly he or she felt about it.

The results were analysed by computer using the Statistical Package for the Social Sciences. Chi-Squares, T tests, tests of proportions and Fisher's exact test were used where applicable. The significance of the results usually influenced decisions about which differences to present. The majority of the statistically significant results presented here satisfied the critical region of 0.05.

In order to understand doctors' attitudes and practices as fully as possible, these professionals were not simply asked about tasks they delegated and for their views on this issue. They were asked, in addition, about their workload, interests, practice organization, work satisfaction, their feelings about the presentation of trivia, and the amount of time available to them to practise their profession.

Some area differences between doctors

Although few differences emerged in terms of the basic characteristics of doctors in this sample and those of doctors as a whole, a number of area differences were found. In particular, the work loads of the doctors varied considerably, as did their degree of work satisfaction. For example, while 10 per cent of doctors in Swansea and 28 per cent of doctors in Newport had list sizes of 3000 patients or more, 33 per cent of doctors interviewed in Croydon and 40 per cent in Kingston had lists of this size. On the other hand, patients in Wales had a higher consulting rate than Kingston, but not Croydon, doctors. While 53 per cent of doctors in Kingston on average saw twenty-one or more patients per surgery, the proportions for Croydon, Swansea and Newport were 100 per cent, 95 per cent, and 94 per cent respectively. Doctors in Kingston were also more likely to say the number of patients seen per surgery was satisfactory, rather than too high – 60 per cent in comparison with 47 per cent in Croydon, 35 per cent in Swansea, and 22 per cent in Newport. Again, satisfaction with general practice was lower in Croydon and Wales than in Kingston. While just 13 per cent of doctors in Kingston said they were not very satisfied with general practice, 21 per cent of doctors in Croydon expressed dissatisfaction with their work, as did 25 per cent of doctors in Swansea and 44 per cent of doctors in Newport. Perhaps the more affluent, middle-class environment of Kingston, in comparison with the other three areas, had some impact on doctors' workloads and satisfaction. Doctors certainly tended to blame the social structure for their problems. For example, of the following two statements, the first was made by a female doctor in a group practice in Kingston and the second was made by a single-handed doctor in Croydon who practised in the middle of a large council housing estate:

> 'I was a GP in Tooting for a while and I felt overworked there. It was a very poor area and patients used to come over such little things. It was demoralizing, they believed it was their right to come. The area where I practise now is totally different. It's very middle class and patients are reluctant to bother you because they're not paying you.'

> 'I see a lot of trivia here where there's a lot of one-parent families and no relatives living nearby to lend a hand. When a child is sick they reach for the phone instead of the sick bowl.'

Delegation patterns and the employment and attachment of ancillary staff also varied according to area. Inevitably, as the extent of delegation depends on the availability of staff to delegate to, these two variables should be closely linked. Significantly, Kingston-on-Thames doctors were more likely to have a treatment room nurse, 47 per cent in comparison with 27 per cent in Croydon, 30 per cent in Swansea and 33 per cent in Newport. Perhaps this may partly explain the lower doctor–patient consulting rate in Kingston, despite higher list sizes, and also the greater amount of satisfaction doctors derived from their work. As would be expected from the variations in the patterns of employment or attachment of treatment room nurses, doctors in Croydon, Swansea, and Newport were more likely to practise no delegation in the surgery at all than doctors in Kingston. The differences can be quantified as 20 per cent, 35 per cent, 28 per cent, and 13 per cent respectively. More doctors in Kingston also possessed favourable attitudes towards the delegation of clinical tasks, 80 per cent in comparison with 53 per cent of Croydon doctors, 65 per cent of Swansea doctors, and 56 per cent of Newport doctors.

What about other ancillary staff? Swansea had the highest rates of attachment and employment of district nurses, health visitors, and administrative staff (receptionists, secretaries, and so on). For example, district nurses were attached to all Swansea doctors interviewed, 94 per cent of Newport doctors, 87 per cent of Croydon doctors and 73 per cent of doctors in Kingston. All Swansea doctors had an attached health visitor in comparison with 94 per cent in Newport, and 73 per cent in both Kingston and Croydon. Finally, 95 per cent of Swansea doctors possessed administrative staff, in comparison with 83 per cent of Newport doctors, 60 per cent of Croydon doctors, and 87 per cent of Kingston doctors. Few doctors in any of the areas had attached social workers and many were confused about the attachment of midwives due to changing attachment policies and the fact that some district nurses were also qualified midwives.

Doctors' perceptions of trivia

'Trivialities are the main problem of general practice. They make life so disheartening. You could be doing something so meaningful but instead you spend your life seeing a lot of rubbish.'

(General practitioner in Wales)

If the presentation of trivial conditions is regarded as a problem by a large proportion of general practitioners, then it could be argued that this supports the case for the greater use of ancillary staff for performing routine medical procedures. On the other hand, it also supports the case for better medical education in general practice with less of a hospital orientation. Doctors' perceptions of trivia are significant as they influence how the general practitioner will define his or her role.

Over half of the doctors interviewed, 54 per cent, felt that the presentation of trivia was a serious problem in general practice. These doctors tended to feel that too many patients presented inappropriate conditions. The doctors expressing this view fell into two categories. The first consisted of doctors who were uninterested in psychiatry and who were less likely to perceive the treatment of emotional problems as within their role. For example, 8 per cent of those questioned in this group expressed a special interest in psychiatry, in comparison with 29 per cent of doctors stating that the presentation of trivia was no problem to them, and 40 per cent felt the treatment of emotional problems was within their role in comparison to 81 per cent of other doctors.

One of the assumptions of doctors who are interested in treating emotional problems is that such problems are often initially presented in the form of a minor physical illness. Thus for these doctors, one of the challenges of general practice is to discover the patient's real reason for the consultation. Doctors uninterested in this branch of medicine are unlikely to respond to this challenge and, because of the hospital ideology they have been socialized into, they see trivial conditions as inappropriately time consuming and therefore a nuisance. This is illustrated by the following two doctors' comments, the first being an elderly man practising from a group in the centre of a Welsh town and the second a middle-aged doctor practising from a group in Surrey:

> 'We have fewer patients to look after these days, but they're far more demanding. We may not do midwifery or suturing any more, but our time is taken up by pill pushers, addicts, people with social problems. Of course, a consultation fee would get rid of some of these.'

> 'Half the patients I saw on Monday morning had nothing wrong with them. I wondered why they had come. On Monday mornings, after the weekend, the place is like Clapham Junction. There are bodies all the way up the stairs. Patients fill the place. If they had to pay two pounds they'd think twice about coming.'

The second category of doctors who felt trivia to be problematic from the doctor's point of view consisted of those with high workloads and who felt that their workloads were too high in terms of the number of patients seen. For example, 63 per cent of these doctors saw twenty-one or more patients per surgery, in comparison with 39 per cent who said trivia was no problem, and 32 per cent performed nine or more home visits daily in comparison with 26 per cent of doctors expressing the latter belief. Also, 81 per cent of doctors complaining about trivia felt they saw too many patients per surgery in comparison with 35 per cent of other doctors and 70 per cent felt their home visiting rate was too high in comparison with 19 per cent of other doctors. These doctors tended to express strong feelings of disillusionment with general practice as the following example shows. This statement was made by an elderly doctor practising from a group in Surrey:

'What is general practice today anyway? It's often a matter of separating the wheat from the chaff. If you excluded a certain 10 per cent of patients in this practice you'd be pushed to do a good day's work.'

Because of the amount of so-called trivial illness seen, doctors often commented that they had lost any expertise or complex skills which they had once possessed. But how did they define trivial conditions? Whether or not non-physicians could deal with such conditions instead of the doctor, or even whether the conditions are regarded as a legitimate part of the doctor's work, partly depends on what these problems are. Trivial conditions were variously defined as social or emotional problems, sore throats, colds and similar ailments. The need for issuing sickness certificates was a further source of irritation. There is undoubtedly a case for the elimination of the present system of sickness certification. In addition, more patient education could reduce the numbers consulting doctors over conditions such as colds. However, in view of the self-limiting nature of many of the conditions presenting in general practice, there is little reason why a non-physician could not screen out and treat minor conditions when they are encountered. More complex cases could be referred to the doctor. Such personnel could also be made aware of the possibility of patients consulting them over emotional problems, camouflaged as physical problems. Any such suspected cases could be referred to the appropriate professional. At the moment it is unclear whether this professional should generally be the doctor.

Does the practice of delegation alter doctors' perceptions of the presentation of trivia as a problem in general practice? The findings of this study indicate that it does not. Doctors who regarded the presentation of trivia as a problem were far more likely than other doctors to delegate a wide range of clinical procedures (at least three of the tasks in *Table 1*), 43 per cent in comparison with 16 per cent. As might be expected, no doctor delegated the initial screening of patients in the surgery so presumably their perceptions of trivia would remain unaffected by the amount of delegation they did practise. But why were doctors practising delegation more likely to see trivia as problematic? Perhaps perceptions of trivia are more dependent upon doctors' personalities than actual workloads. This suggests that at present it is intolerance of patient behaviour that leads doctors to delegate medical procedures, rather than a desire to improve the quality and efficiency of general practice. This may explain why over two-thirds, 70 per cent, of the doctors who felt trivia to be a problem wanted to see consultation fees introduced as a deterrent to patients seeking help for minor ailments. In comparison, just under a third, 32 per cent, of other doctors wanted to see consultation fees introduced.

What are the implications for the future role of the general practitioner? It does not appear that a large majority of general practitioners want to concentrate more on emotional problems as this was one of the most frequent examples of trivia given. Moreover, a mere 59 per cent felt the treatment of such problems came within their role and many of these said this was simply because there was no one else to treat them. Perhaps clinical medicine is preferred? However, just 25 per cent arranged for ECGs to be undertaken in their practices and 34 per cent cervical smears. Only 12 per cent of the doctors interviewed performed minor surgery regularly in their practices and 19 per cent occasionally. However, 69 per cent of doctors were willing to undertake more of the minor work presently done by accident and emergency departments if they had more time and better facilities, and if they were offered financial incentives. The practice of more complex clinical medicine might increase doctors' satisfaction with their work and reduce feelings of frustration. If this is to happen, the practice of delegation, enabling doctors to develop and extend their work, becomes more important.

Doctors' perceptions of time available

'Many patients don't need more time devoted to them as most consultations are unnecessary anyway. But because so many people consult over trivia it means I can't devote sufficient time to those patients who may have a serious condition.'

(General practitioner in Surrey)

Sixty-two per cent of doctors felt they had insufficient time to devote to patients whom they felt needed their attention. Of those who felt the presentation of trivia constituted a problem, 84 per cent also felt time was a problem, in comparison with 35 per cent of those not feeling trivia to be a problem.

Doctors who believed that time was a problem fell into two main categories. The first consisted of those who were less interested in psychiatry and who were less likely to see the treatment of emotional problems as within their role. For example, 10 per cent of doctors who felt time to be a problem were interested in psychiatry in comparison with 31 per cent who felt time was no problem; and 50 per cent of doctors who felt time to be a problem felt the treatment of emotional problems fell within their role, in comparison with 73 per cent of other doctors. As with the question of trivia, personality factors also possibly affect doctors' perceptions of time available.

Practice situations seemed likely to affect doctors' perceptions of time as a problem. The second main category consisted of doctors who saw more patients per surgery and who performed more home visits than doctors not perceiving time as a problem. For example, 57 per cent of doctors feeling time to be a problem saw twenty-one or more patients per surgery, in comparison with 42 per cent of other doctors; also 38 per cent performed nine or more home visits daily in comparison with 15 per cent of others. Doctors who saw time as a problem were more likely to feel they saw too many patients per surgery, 95 per cent in comparison with 4 per cent of others, and were also more likely to practise in Wales than in England, 67 per cent in comparison with 38 per cent. South Wales, where two of the study areas are situated, has a higher morbidity and patient consulting rate than South-East England where the other two study areas are located (Tudor Hart 1976). Under such conditions, it is not surprising that doctors seeing time as problematic expressed less satisfaction with general practice. Thirty-three per cent of doctors feeling this expressed a low degree of satisfaction in comparison with 15 per cent of those not seeing time as a problem.

Many doctors attributed their problems with time to the system of remuneration. For example, one elderly Welsh doctor, who practised alone, commented:

> 'My major grumble is that we're not able to give a good service because we haven't the time. You have to take on too many patients to live, and you have to do outside work to live.'

Apart from changing the present capitation system of remuneration, this statement could be used as a strong argument in favour of an increased amount of delegation. However, no relationship was found between doctors' perceptions of time as a problem and the amount of delegation practised. Possibly, as suggested earlier, delegation is not being practised as efficiently as it could be.

The extent of delegation to nurses in general practice

> 'Nurses could do much more but we doctors tend to be very conservative. We complain of having too much work but we're very reluctant to delegate any of it.'
>
> (General practitioner in Surrey)

Many of the doctors interviewed occasionally delegated minor clinical procedures to nurses, but far fewer delegated them regularly. *Table 1* shows, for example, that in no case did the proportion delegating any minor clinical task regularly exceed 43 per cent. Doctors who regularly delegated three or more of the six procedures listed in the table were classified as practising a high degree of delegation. Doctors who delegated one or two of the procedures regularly or occasionally, or who delegated three or more but only occasionally, were classified as practising a low degree of delegation. Thirty-one per cent of doctors practised a high degree of delegation according to this classification, 44 per cent practised a low degree and 25 per cent practised no delegation in the surgery at all.

Table 1   *Frequency of delegation of minor clinical tasks in surgery*

	Frequency with which procedure is delegated:			Number of doctors
	regularly	occasionally	never	
injections, dressings, suture removal	38%	31%	31%	
immunizations and vaccinations	32%	16%	52%	
ear syringing	43%	19%	38%	68
venepuncture	19%	15%	66%	
cervical cytology	4%	4%	92%	
minor surgical tasks e.g. incision of boils	—	—	100%	

Source: Bowling, A. (1980). Nurses in the Primary Care Team.
Lancet **ii**: 590. Reprinted with permission.

Doctors practising a high degree of delegation differed in a number of ways from other doctors, as *Table 2* shows. For example, they were more likely to practise from a group of doctors, to be more recent medical graduates and to undertake a wider range of medical procedures and activities. They were also more likely to have a higher degree of practice organization, measured by the possession of a treatment room nurse (practice nurse) and an appointment system.

Although it was previously suggested that delegation might affect workload patterns (the number of patients seen by doctors) and also levels of satisfaction that doctors derive from their work, no differences between these variables were found. Perhaps this is because doctors do not practise delegation efficiently or extensively enough.

Table 2　*The extent of delegation and differences between doctors*

	Proportion of doctors practising:		
	a high degree of delegation in surgery	a low degree of delegation in surgery	no delegation in surgery
practices with three or more doctors	90%	57%	18%
graduated 1960 or later	48%	23%	23%
technical procedures are performed in the practice, such as cervical cytology; electro-cardiography (ECG); haemoglobin levels (HB); erythrocyte sediment-ation rate (ESR)	81%	40%	12%
holds special clinics	71%	50%	24%
has part-time hospital appointment	48%	10%	24%
has special medical interest (excluding psychiatry)	48%	43%	12%
has a full appointment system	90%	70%	24%
has a practice nurse or nurse/receptionist	100%	7%	—
Number of doctors (=100%)	21	30	17

Attitudes towards delegating clinical procedures

'My policy is if you want anything done well do it yourself.'
(General practitioner in Wales)

The proportion of doctors not delegating particular tasks regularly at present but who were in favour of doing so ranged from 49 per cent to 62 per cent depending on the task. These proportions are disappointing in view of the simple nature of the clinical tasks asked about. For example, of those doctors not regularly delegating injections, dressings, and suture removal regularly in the surgery, 62 per cent held favourable attitudes towards their regular delegation. Of those not delegating immunizations and vaccinations regularly, 54 per cent held favourable attitudes on this issue. Forty-nine per cent of those not regularly delegating ear syringing were in favour of so doing. The comparable proportions for venepuncture, cervical cytology and minor surgery were 58 per cent, 49 per cent and 62 per cent respectively. As *Table 1* showed, no doctor at present delegated minor surgical tasks either regularly or occasionally. Taking those doctors not delegating particular procedures either regularly or occasionally in the surgery, in no instance would more than half of these doctors have been willing to delegate them regularly in the future. A small number of doctors initially expressing favourable attitudes towards delegation would not have been willing to practise delegation themselves.

In order to analyse doctors' attitudes more closely on this issue, they were divided into two groups. The first group included those in favour of delegating at least four of the six listed clinical tasks. These were then classified as doctors favouring delegation. The second group included doctors not in favour of delegating any procedure, and those not in favour of delegating more than three of the six groups of tasks. These comprised the group with unfavourable attitudes. Sixty-three per cent of doctors were included in the first group and 37 per cent in the second.

Apart from the relevance of the year of graduation, 40 per cent of doctors with favourable attitudes graduated in 1960 or later in comparison with 16 per cent of other doctors; on the whole doctors with favourable attitudes fell into two groups. First, they tended to have a broader conception of their technical role and to have more specialist interests. For example, 58 per cent of them had arrangements in their surgeries for undertaking technical procedures such as cervical cytology, electrocardiography, and the recording of haemoglobin levels and erythrocyte sedimentation rates. In contrast, a mere 24 per cent of the group with unfavourable attitudes towards delegation had made such arrangements. Thirty-three per cent of the first group held a part-time hospital appointment, in comparison with only 12 per cent of those with unfavourable attitudes. Finally, 58 per cent held special clinics in their surgeries in comparison with 36 per cent of other doctors, and 60 per cent had postgraduate qualifications in contrast to 24 per cent of the unfavourable group.

Second, doctors with favourable attitudes were more likely to have attempted some degree of organization within their practices. For example, 77 per cent had a full appointment system in contrast to 44 per cent of doctors with unfavourable attitudes, and 44 per cent had a treatment room nurse in comparison with 16 per cent of other doctors. They were also more likely to practise with three or more doctors, 63 per cent in comparison with 48 per cent.

It appears, then, that practice organization and the range of medical activities undertaken are related both to the amount of delegation practised and to doctors' attitudes towards delegation. It was suggested earlier that doctors with a broader conception of their role would perhaps feel less threatened by delegation. A stronger emphasis in medical education on broadening doctors' perceptions of their role and on improving practice efficiency may create a more favourable environment for the encouragement of delegation and patterns of delegation may expand as a new generation of less conservative doctors emerges.

Reasons given by doctors for their attitudes towards delegation

'I entered general practice because it offered the opportunity to do what I wanted, to be my own boss. I can do this by remaining single handed and by doing everything myself.'

(General practitioner in Wales)

On the whole, doctors mentioned three types of advantages and four types of disadvantages resulting from the delegation of clinical tasks. For example, 49 per cent said that delegation saves the doctor's time. As two young doctors practising from groups in Surrey said:

'I don't enjoy doing minor procedures. I don't go along with the argument that putting a bandage on a patient's sprained ankle gives you more contact with your patient. It's time consuming and the nurse is better at it than me.'

'Younger doctors are beginning to realize that there's so much more you can do with general practice given the time. I didn't do biochemistry to spend my life syringing ears.'

Far fewer, 16 per cent, mentioned that delegation results in a better distribution of skills, and only 18 per cent noted that delegation enhances the doctor's satisfaction with work. No doctor mentioned the effect delegation has on the role and work satisfaction of the nurse, the person tasks are usually delegated to. It is this lack of consideration which often leads to friction between doctors and nursing organizations.

Not all doctors with favourable attitudes towards delegation were able to delegate as much as they wished. One recent immigrant, who practised with one other doctor, relied on the district nurse to perform delegated clinical tasks when she had time. He felt frustrated by the limitations this reliance imposed upon him, although he had not considered employing his own nurse to work in the surgery:

'Of course a nurse should do all these minor procedures. What on earth do doctors do biochemistry for? Not to spend their lives syringing ears.

Nurses even do anaesthetics in America, and in Sweden – everywhere except here! There's no need for GPs to be academically qualified in this country. A nurse could do 60 per cent of my work. You don't need GPs in this country. GPs don't use their training.'

Fifteen per cent of doctors who wanted to delegate tasks to a nurse said they were unable to do so because they had no treatment room nurse and the district nurses attached to their practices were not permitted to undertake delegated tasks. None of these doctors had considered the possibility of employing their own nurses to work in a treatment room. They failed to appreciate that the district nurse's primary obligations are to community nursing, not surgery work. This attitude is evident in the following young Welsh doctor's comment. Although this doctor practised from a health centre he had no treatment room nurse:

> 'I'm all in favour of delegation. The problem is the district nurse is only here for a while in the mornings. It's fine if a patient comes in when she's arrived and wants his ears syringed. I can say "Go and see the nurse". But I usually do such things myself as she's not here all the time. This is a nuisance.'

In view of such restrictions it is not surprising that even doctors with attached nurses are increasingly employing their own nurses (Reedy, Philips, and Newell 1976). The restrictions imposed by the area health authorities on the use of district nurses for treatment room work often led to feelings of resentment in those doctors who wanted to practise delegation but had no treatment room nurse to delegate to. For example, another young Welsh doctor who had unsuccessfully attempted to persuade his attached district nurse to perform clinical tasks in the surgery said:

> 'Venepuncture, ear syringing, injections, dressings and so on are very time-consuming things for us. All these are simple enough procedures. I think the arguments put forward by the AHA that they don't want nurses doing some of these things because of legal problems are really just excuses. Really they don't want them extensively used by us.'

Eighteen per cent of doctors said they would like to delegate tasks to a nurse, but had no practice facilities or space for a nurse to work in. The increasing development of health centres, and the improvement of existing premises, may help to overcome this problem. However, only five of the doctors interviewed practised from a health centre, and only seven, in reply to a direct question, said they would like to. The remainder felt that health centres were too expensive to maintain, that they would lose their independence if they practised from one, and that they would lose control over ancillary staff who would usually be employed by the area health authority.

Two doctors, although keen to delegate, felt resentful that they had to take legal responsibility for the actions of the nurse. For example, as one of them said:

> 'One thing is nurses won't take responsibility for their own actions. This is ridiculous. They must have some skills, they're trained nurses, why won't they use them? The problem with nurses is that they're obsessed with defining what their role is. This is the biggest problem. Why can't they just get on with the job?'

Not all doctors held favourable attitudes towards delegation. The opposition towards this concept expressed by some doctors was formidable.

For example, 35 per cent of doctors indicated that they believed delegation threatens the independence of the doctor. Only 4 per cent of these doctors had graduated since 1960, in comparison with 46 per cent of other doctors. As previously argued, older doctors probably define independence more rigidly and regard teamwork as alien to this concept. It may be difficult to alter the attitudes and practices of earlier graduates who have had longer experiences of unaided practice. As one elderly, single-handed doctor in an affluent part of Surrey said:

> 'I don't want anyone interfering in my practice. I prefer to work completely on my own. You're more independent this way. I don't even like working with other doctors. I can see younger doctors may be more willing to look at this delegation more seriously, but GPs of my age group are too insular. The thing is, general practice was the first career choice for many doctors in my day because it meant you really were an independent practitioner. We tend to equate independence and clinical freedom with the freedom to do exactly what we want with no interference.'

Doctors expressing such views also tended to reveal some degree of conservatism in their attitudes. Seventy-five per cent of the doctors who believe delegation threatens their independence made statements reflecting this. One example is the statement made by a middle-aged doctor, practising with two others, in Wales:

> 'We don't delegate anything . . . the thing is I've been doing these things for donkey's years and I've just continued to do them. When I first started I was on my own, no receptionist or anything. I'm too old to change now.'

The implication seems to be that there will be little progress over delegation until older doctors are replaced by more recent graduates.

Twenty-six per cent of doctors felt that delegation does not save the doctor's time, but simply creates more work because of the general incompetence of ancillary staff. These doctors expressed misgivings about the abilities of anyone other than a fully trained doctor. For example, one older Welsh doctor who practised from a partnership of two said:

> 'I do all the ear syringing, everything in fact. If you ask someone else to do things they will invariably be cocked up.'

These doctors felt that ancillary staff merely 'get under your feet' and create more work by 'consulting you all the time'. When they were asked for their views of either further-trained nurses or specially trained assistants performing the clinical tasks in question, negative views were again expressed. One such doctor, an elderly woman practising in Surrey, worked alone from extremely dilapidated premises. While the author was waiting to see the doctor patients appeared to be waiting up to two hours in a room so crowded that there was no space for many of them to sit down. However, this doctor still denied the necessity for ancillary staff and insisted on performing every procedure herself. She had little contact with the district nurse and health visitor attached to her practice and even performed dressings herself:

> 'I've worked alone here for forty years. My surgeries are crowded every day but I can manage perfectly well on my own. I don't want to start delegating and I don't need to. I don't want any ancillary help. They would just get under your feet. They don't help you do more work, nor even relieve you. All they do is talk.'

Twenty-two per cent of doctors were reluctant to delegate minor clinical procedures because they believed them to be within the legitimate role of the doctor. Narrow conceptions of the role of the nurse also tended to be held: 'A doctor does a doctor's work and a nurse does a nurse's work, which is bathing and dressing.' There were indications that doctors maintained these procedures were part of their role because they felt threatened. The following statement by a Welsh doctor, working in a three-man practice, who initially held positive attitudes towards delegation provides an example of this feeling of threat:

> 'But what would I do instead if I delegated all this? I really think, after all, that these procedures should remain in the doctor's province.'

These doctors often commented that minor procedures were the legitimate domain of the doctor because they helped doctors to build up a relationship with patients. A middle-aged Welsh doctor practising with just one other said:

> 'You know relationships between people don't happen instantaneously. They're the result of a collection of small events. A minor procedure such as ear syringing can seal that relationship. It's the doctor–patient relationship that's so important. That's why these procedures are really the doctor's job.'

Altogether, 16 per cent of doctors mentioned the doctor–patient relationship as a reason for not wanting to practise delegation. It was felt that delegation, by the introduction of a third person, would form a barrier between doctor and patient. The concept of personal doctoring was taken literally. However, no one mentioned in this context the fact that, due to lack of time, there was often little opportunity to develop this relationship anyway.

Doctors mentioning the doctor–patient relationship tended to be earlier graduates than other doctors, 82 per cent graduated before 1950 in comparison with 32 per cent of other doctors, and they tended to practise alone or with only one other doctor, 82 per cent in comparison with 35 per cent of other doctors. If older doctors are more likely to value their independence, as has been suggested, they may be more likely to perceive delegation as a threat in a further sense: interference with the doctor–patient relationship. The doctor–patient relationship may be regarded as a symbol of the doctor's independence, and also as the essence of general practice. To suggest innovations which may be perceived as threatening that relationship could be seen as threatening the essence and independent position of general practice itself. Consequently, such innovations are likely to be opposed.

Other findings also suggest that doctors mentioning the doctor–patient relationship in this context may not always have had the best interests of the patient in mind. For example, there was no significant difference between these and other doctors on the issue of attitudes towards the introduction of a consultation fee. In each case, approximately half the doctors were in favour of such a fee. It would not be expected that doctors concerned about the quality of their relationships with patients would want such fees, as they impose a financial barrier between doctor and patient. It could alternatively be argued that financial constraints to consulting lead to doctors seeing fewer patients and thus enables them to spend more time with each patient.

In this sense, a financial barrier may enhance the doctor–patient relationship for the few for whom financial outlays are of little consequence, but what about the majority?

It would also be expected that doctors mentioning the doctor–patient relationship would be more concerned about treating the 'whole person'. However, there was no difference between these and other doctors in perceptions of the doctor's role in the treatment of emotional problems. Just over half in each case thought treatment of such problems was within the doctor's role. Nor were doctors mentioning this relationship more likely to hold clinics other than normal surgeries in their practices or to perform a wider range of medical procedures – methods of practice which might enhance the doctor–patient relationship by obviating the need for referral to hospital. For example, about half of each group of doctors held special clinics, about a fifth of doctors mentioning the doctor–patient relationship performed minor surgery in their practices in comparison with a third of other doctors, and fewer, approximately a fifth, arranged for technical procedures to be carried out on their premises in comparison with just over a half of other doctors (for example, cervical cytology, ECG, ESR, HB).

Doctors stating that delegation threatens the doctor–patient relationship appeared to be more afraid of losing any part of this relationship to non-physicians than actually valuing the quality of the relationship itself. As has been pointed out previously, the general practitioner has been largely excluded from hospital medicine, but has retained the patient. Thus, some doctors, particularly those who have experienced the role and status insecurity inherent in the history of general practice, will be reluctant to accept organizational changes which might further remove the patient from them. This insecurity, in addition to narrow definitions of independence particularly apparent among older doctors, may limit the amount of delegation practised.

Two other reasons for reluctance to delegate either at all or extensively were mentioned by a small number of doctors: fear of legal problems and the system of remuneration. Concerning remuneration, the issue of delegation may have economic implications for some doctors. In Britain a limited fee per item of service system of remuneration operates alongside the capitation system in general practice. Doctors receive additional payments for procedures such as the insertion of intrauterine devices, immunizations and vaccinations, cervical cytology, and the prescription of the contraceptive pill. As a few doctors pointed out, the performance of such procedures supplements their incomes and it is possible that ancillary staff would start requesting part of this additional remuneration if such tasks were delegated to them. One doctor who practised with three others from large purpose-built premises in Wales said:

> 'I don't go along with all this talk of delegation. You have to bear in mind the in-roads this could have on the income of doctors. These procedures do supplement our income quite considerably, and our income is quite tight as it is.'

Seventy-two per cent of doctors, in response to an earlier question, said they would like to see the system altered to a complete fee-for-service system. However, this may act as a disincentive to delegation for the previously noted reason. Since the item-for-service system of remuneration is limited in this country, experience indicates that without it doctors neither delegate nor perform many procedures themselves. Many doctors noted that the removal of a sebaceous cyst, for example, takes at least half and hour and involves the use of materials which doctors have to provide out of their own incomes.

A significant minority of doctors held negative attitudes towards the delegation of clinical tasks. Perhaps medical educators need to adopt a more positive attitude towards delegation if doctors' prejudices are to be overcome, although this prejudice was more blatant among earlier graduates. Nevertheless, doctors could still be taught that delegation does not necessarily lead to a usurpation of their power and independence, or to an encroachment upon their role. Before the latter can be taught, however, the role of the general practitioner needs to be clearly defined. Then doctors can unequivocally be taught that delegation may free them to concentrate upon their medical skills, perhaps even enhancing their satisfaction with their work. But what of the delegation of diagnostic procedures? How do general practitioners view this?

The delegation of initial home visits

> 'The delegation of home visits would be great . . . then we could spend from nine till five in the surgery. We'd have much more time to spend with the patients who consulted us.'
>
> (General practitioner in Wales)

Doctors were asked whether they ever delegated initial home visits whereby nurses decided whether a doctor's visit was necessary. None of the doctors interviewed delegated such visits on a regular basis, although 23 per cent delegated them occasionally. Perhaps not surprisingly, these doctors were more likely to be satisfied with their home-visiting rate, 75 per cent in comparison with 46 per cent of other doctors.

The delegation of initial home visiting is a controversial issue. None of the divisional or area nursing officers in the study areas approved of their nurses undertaking such visits. Despite this, 89 per cent of the doctors delegating such visits delegated them to attached community nursing staff.

Forty-four per cent of all doctors interviewed were in favour of the regular delegation of initial home visits, and 90 per cent of these said they would delegate them regularly given suitable staff. Again, doctors with favourable attitudes were more likely to find the presentation of trivia a problem in general practice, 67 per cent in comparison with 45 per cent of other doctors.

It would be expected that the delegation of such visits would be more controversial among doctors, especially as only 26 per cent were in favour of such initial screening assessments being made in the surgery, and only 15 per cent were in favour of a non-physician simply preparing each patient and taking a brief medical history before calling in the doctor. Moreover, only 15 per cent of doctors would actually have been willing to delegate initial screening in the surgery themselves, and only 12 per cent would have been willing to delegate the initial preparation of patients. It appears that it is mainly in the surgery that the doctor is unwilling to forgo the role of person of first contact. Perhaps there is less kudos attached to home visiting. Most doctors proudly announced that they had cut their home-visiting rates over the past few years. However, the reason usually given for their reluctance to make home visits was that they were too time consuming. As one young Surrey doctor said:

> 'I don't mind so much seeing patients over trivial complaints in the surgery as in the home as it doesn't take up so much time. Home calls take time.'

The delegation of initial screening in the surgery

> 'I think this concept is very viable, but I can see why a lot of doctors will be opposed to it. If you take away the trivia what will we do all day? Trivia occupies the bulk of our workload, we thrive on it.'
>
> (General practitioner in Surrey)

Doctors were also asked about their attitudes towards the introduction of physicians' assistants or nurse practitioners to initially screen patients in the surgery. The purpose of such screening was explained:

to decide which patients needed to be seen by the doctor and which could be treated by non-physicians. As expected, most doctors were opposed to this concept. Twenty-six per cent of the doctors interviewed were in favour of it but only 15 per cent would have been willing to delegate such initial screening themselves. Those in favour, but who would not practise it themselves, saw advantages only for larger practices. For example, an elderly single-handed doctor in Wales said:

> 'I can see that these people are needed in some practices. They would be an excellent idea in large health centres for example, but not here, not in my practice. As long as they don't affect me that's all right.'

Doctors in favour of initial screening were more likely to be delegating to a high degree already. For example, 45 per cent practised a high degree of delegation in comparision with 26 per cent of other doctors. They were also more likely than other doctors to delegate initial home visits, 50 per cent in comparison with 14 per cent. Again, they were more likely to see trivia as a problem, 78 per cent in comparison with 46 per cent of doctors with unfavourable attitudes. It is difficult to speculate on the basis of these findings whether it is intolerance of patient behaviour which encourages doctors to delegate and to hold favourable attitudes towards various types of delegation, or whether the practice of delegation leads to favourable attitudes. There were no indications, in the case of initial screening, that the gradual replacement of older doctors by more recent graduates would alter the situation, as no significant differences with age were found.

When asked about the type of personnel initial screening could be delegated to, 55 per cent of those in favour of the concept said they would prefer to delegate this to a nurse with further training and 17 per cent said they would prefer to delegate to a nurse as presently trained. Twenty-eight per cent said they would prefer a specially trained physician's assistant to perform this function. The majority, then, preferred to delegate to a familiar figure, a nurse. Nurses may often be seen as less threatening. A recent entrant to general practice in a Surrey group said:

> 'I'd rather a nurse undertook this screening role. The introduction of physicians' assistants may lead to a lot of interference.'

The main advantage of initial screening referred to by doctors was the saving of the doctor's time. This was mentioned by 22 per cent. A small number said that such a method of organization would result in a better distribution of skills and would enhance the degree of satisfaction they derived from their work.

However, the majority of doctors were opposed to the concept of initial screening in the surgery by a non-physician. This is not unexpected, as various reports on general practice have unanimously declared the general practitioner to be the professional of first contact in the British health service. The immediate reaction of most doctors interviewed was to dismiss initial screening with no prior thought, and only later was an attempt made to justify their responses. A typical comment was: 'It's a diabolical idea'. Eight main reasons were given for negative attitudes towards such screening.

Fifty-one per cent said that a doctor should remain the person of first clinical contact because only fully qualified doctors could diagnose. However, 57 per cent of these doctors felt trivia was a problem in general practice and 63 per cent saw time as a problem. Why then did they react so negatively towards a concept aimed at giving them more time and reducing the number of less complex cases seen? Why did they feel that only doctors should diagnose? Some appeared to genuinely believe that only doctors could safely diagnose: 'There's always the danger of further complications which could be missed'. Many doctors' statements, on the other hand, reflected feelings of role insecurity and role threat: 'The doctor's job is to diagnose, you can't really delegate it'. And as one elderly, single-handed practitioner in Surrey said:

> 'I feel that patients ought to see the doctor first. The doctor should be the first contact. The whole point of general practice is to distinguish the complex from the simple. This screening is the job of the doctor, not someone semi-qualified.'

Such statements were similar to those made by doctors who explicitly said that the introduction of intermediaries for initial screening would obviate the need for fully qualified doctors. This may be an increasing fear at a time of threatened doctor unemployment and 10 per cent of doctors expressed this fear. For example, one elderly doctor in Surrey, who practised with one other doctor, was extremely cynical about the work of the general practitioner:

> 'I can see that much of the work of the GP will eventually be taken over by someone with less training. Of course, one of the problems with this, and even more so if a physician's assistant was introduced instead, is that I'd be done out of a job then. GPs are no more than physicians' assistants these days. The work is very repetitive and untechnical. After a few years in practice you forget any skills you once had.'

Thus while some argued that diagnosis is too complex to delegate, others argued that, in general practice, it demanded few skills as most consultations were for such minor ailments, hence the feeling of role threat: 'If we introduced physicians' assistants here we may as well not bother to train doctors'.

Nineteen per cent of doctors felt the physician should remain the first contact as only they could recognize emotional problems, which may be camouflaged by trivial complaints. This concept is related to that of the drug doctor, as previously pointed out, and maintains that doctors should concern themselves with treating emotional problems. It is believed that the doctor, by acting as counsellor, can be the therapeutic agent. Some doctors think that one of the means by which general practitioners can develop a body of knowledge, thus enhancing their professional status, is by concentration upon this branch of medicine. Such doctors may see initial screening by non-physicians as a potential threat to this aspect of their role. One young Surrey doctor, who practised from a group and who also held a - London teaching hospital appointment, was acutely aware of this issue. He was atypical of most doctors in that he had given much thought to the nurse practitioner/physician's assistant movement in the United States prior to being contacted by the author:

> 'I'm worried about the effects physicians' assistants may have on doctors themselves. It might make them even more redundant. Medical care is increasingly becoming useless as Illich has pointed out, and patients are realizing this. The status of the doctor is declining now as people realize it was sanitation, not drugs, that overcame disease. I feel the introduction of physicians' assistants or nurse practitioners would lower the status of the GP even more by showing how dispensable he is. I believe our efforts should be concentrated upon general practice before we lose it altogether. We must use GPs properly. I believe we should encourage people to go to their GPs with emotional problems. This is where the GP could make a real contribution, and this is where screening would be a disadvantage as people may consult over a minor complaint but it really covers up some major emotional problem they need to talk about and receive advice over. Such complex problems need very highly trained doctors to cope with them. Good medicine needs to be practised by those with a very high level of training. Nurse practitioners and physicians' assistants would form a barrier here.'

As would be expected, all doctors arguing that only they could recognize emotional problems believed that the treatment of such problems was within their role, in comparison with 51 per cent of other doctors. They were also more likely to mention a special interest in psychiatry, 46 per cent in comparison with 11 per cent. These doctors had clearly been influenced by Balint's (1957) work. They gave examples of consultations such as: 'I find a woman uses her child as an excuse to come', 'Emotional problems are really what they've come for, not the headache they tell you about initially', 'The patient with backache may really have a sexual problem.' As the following statement, made by the previously quoted Surrey doctor, shows, doctors interested in emotional problems are not always solely motivated by concern for the patient. Professional interests also intervene:

> 'I don't think the concept of the physician's assistant is applicable to our system. After all in America they were introduced because of the lack of generalists. Here we have a system in which the general practitioner is the backbone of the whole health service. I have reservations about this screening idea . . . especially as general practice is taking a bit of a bashing now anyway. I'm one of the newer schools of thought who are trying to make general practice a specialty in its own right, and one of the foundations of general practice is the doctor–patient relationship. I think the future of general practice lies in concentration upon patients' emotional problems, and the successful treatment of such problems depends upon the establishment of a good doctor–patient relationship. The use of intermediaries to initially screen patients would lead to a less personal system of care. It would lead to more barriers between doctors and patients. This would be to the detriment, not only of the patient, but also of general practice. General practice would become just clinical medicine with no distinctive features of its own.'

Even when doctors are primarily interested in clinical medicine the doctor–patient relationship may be viewed as a central feature of general practice. For example, 30 per cent of all doctors said they felt the introduction of intermediaries for screening purposes would impose a barrier between doctor and patient and adversely affect the doctor–patient relationship. Most of these doctors practised alone or with one other doctor, 71 per cent in comparison with 30 per cent of other doctors. As previously indicated, these doctors often choose to practise in this way in order to retain as much independence as possible. For them, the doctor–patient relationship symbolizes that independence. As before, other findings indicate that it is not always the quality of this relationship that doctors are concerned about. Rather, they are afraid of losing any part of it to members of another profession. For example, doctors mentioning the doctor–patient relationship in this context were no less likely to want to see consultation fees introduced, 50 per cent in comparison with 50 per cent of other doctors. Nor were they any more likely to perform minor surgical procedures for patients; rather than referring them to hospital, 19 per cent performed them in comparison with 38 per cent of other doctors. Further, they were no more likely to arrange for the various technical tasks to be performed on their premises (such as smears, ECG, HB, and ESR). Thirty-eight per cent made such arrangements in contrast to 49 per cent of other doctors. These latter differences were not statistically significant. To some extent, these findings lend support to belief that doctors' feelings of threat are hidden by symbols of caring (McKnight 1977). Admittedly, many doctors had commendable motives when raising the issue of the doctor–patient relationship. For example, one doctor in his late fifties, practising from a two-man partnership in Surrey, said:

> 'I like to see each of my patients in order to build up a relationship with them. Screening would really get rid of the personal doctor. I don't think patients would like this, nor would I. Half of medicine is communicating and advising.'

On the other hand, he clearly also felt threatened, as well as considering his patients' feelings. He does not want his personal doctoring role infringed upon. Such views are understandable in view of the general practitioner's history of role and status insecurity.

As with the delegation of clinical tasks, 35 per cent said they thought the introduction of an intermediary to initially screen patients would threaten their independence. These doctors tended to be earlier graduates, 63 per cent graduated before 1950 in contrast to 27 per cent of other doctors. They tended to express preferences to work with little or no ancillary help: 'I think general practice is great. You're your own boss. I make the decisions', 'I'm free to do what I want, when I want. This is important to me'. Doctors expressing this view often practised alone or with only one other doctor, 54 per cent in comparison with 39 per cent of other doctors. The following state- ment by a Welsh doctor shows the relationship between the older doctor who entered general practice because it offered a degree of independence and who has remained single handed for that reason. The doctor–patient relationship can be seen as symbolizing that independence:

> 'I don't doubt that a well-trained nurse could cope quite well screening patients first, but I would not like a filter system in my practice. I just wouldn't be happy unless I saw every patient. I like to get to know each of my patients personally. A filter system would act as a barrier in this respect. I entered general practice because it offered the opportunity to do what I want, to be my own boss. By remaining single handed I can provide a personal service for my patients. Doctors working in small

practices like this prefer the personal aspects of practice, with few other
staff to come between them and their patients.'

Doctors feeling their independence would be threatened by intermediaries expressed distrust of ancillaries generally: 'Of course,
health visitors are the damn nuisance here', 'And as for social
workers . . . . It's all very well in theory, but people don't want them
poking their noses in', 'When a nurse . . . screens first . . . the nurse
would begin to attach more importance to her role than her training
warranted', 'Patients still don't know what health visitors and social
workers are yet'. Possibly some doctors must share the blame for the
latter situation. Such statements indicate that experiments with
initial screening may have to be postponed until a new generation of
less conservative doctors emerges.

Thirteen per cent of doctors argued that the introduction of intermediaries for screening purposes would lower the standard of medical
care. However, these doctors were no less likely than other doctors to
delegate initial home visits, 33 per cent and 22 per cent respectively.
Nor were they any less likely to be in favour of their delegation, in each
case 44 per cent were in favour. Doctors' views on initial screening in
the surgery and in the home appear to be inconsistent. They clearly
experience less threat by other professionals taking over home visits
for initial assessment purposes. Perhaps this is because they are not
regarded as such a central part of the doctor's role, and are merely
seen as time consuming.

The feeling that screening in the surgery would lower standards
may often be based on a fear of role encroachment. It is based on the
assumption that there is a relationship between our presently organized system of medical care, with doctors possessing full autonomy,
and high-quality medical care. One young Welsh doctor inadvert-
ently appeared to allude to the crux of the issue when discussing direct
access to hospital facilities:

> 'We have direct access to everything except bone and joint X-rays and
> sinus X-rays. This is a nuisance as direct access saves us so much time.
> The problem is they don't want to let go of what they have.'

Great power lies in the doctor's right to the prerogative of deciding
upon the question, or diagnosis. It may be expected that doctors
would regard the delegation of this aspect of medicine as leading to
'second-rate care'. One individual, an elderly Surrey doctor who
practised entirely alone, without even a receptionist, had a particularly high opinion of his quality:

'I disapprove of that (screening) entirely. It's like not allowing everyone to see the Duke of Edinburgh or the Queen.'

Thirty per cent of doctors opposed initial screening because they felt it would not save their time. They felt that ancillary staff would merely 'get under your feet' and 'just encourage another hundred patients to come'. Some of these doctors expressed the view that patients should be discouraged from attending the surgery at all over minor complaints. One doctor suggested that the chemist should be permitted to prescribe for minor ailments: 'That's my solution. Not a nurse practitioner or whatever you call them, but the chemist.'

Finally, 28 per cent of doctors said that a system of initial screening should not be introduced as 'patients would not like it'. However, 68 per cent of these doctors were in favour of the introduction of a consultation fee in comparison with 47 per cent of other doctors. Patients' feelings were not considered here. Overall, doctors tended to feel that patients would not accept such a system, not because it might be of low quality, but because they expect to see the most highly trained personnel available: doctors. 'They come to see the doctor, no one else.' The validity of the argument about non-acceptance by patients is questionable. No doubt if such a system were introduced without careful explanation to patients it would not be accepted. Patient acceptance may often depend on doctor acceptance. As two Welsh doctors, both practising from groups of three, said:

'Patients have found referral to the nurse quite acceptable. This is probably because we approve. Their attitudes are governed by the doctor's attitudes.'

'There's no problem of patient acceptance of nurses in casualty, and the casualty sister often runs the place. This is probably because we accept this and they're used to seeing the nurse there.'

Summary and discussion

Although many doctors found the presentation of trivia in the surgery to be a problem, and although many also felt they did not have enough time to spend with patients who needed their attention, strong resistance towards the delegation of even simple clinical tasks was found among a significant minority of doctors. Doctors were even less receptive towards the delegation of tasks more clearly within their role, such as diagnosis. However, it appears from this study that, at least with regard to the delegation of clinical procedures, as more doctors practise from groups, and take more interest in efficient methods of practice organization and in undertaking a wider range of medical procedures and activities, then more extensive delegation may ensue. These changes may occur as more recent graduates replace older doctors and as they become discontent with misutilizing their skills, a discontent which may be expressed in terms of frustration with trivia. However, at present there is little point in encouraging delegation until some of the features of the present organization of general practice have been eroded. The concept of an expanded nurse role, or even of a physician's assistant, is not logical in a country where single-handed or small group practices predominate. There is no future for the reallocation of tasks within the health team if no health team exists.

Resistance to delegation was expressed largely in terms of feelings of threat to independence and professionalism and fears of role encroachment. Such attitudes are understandable. Traditionally, the general practitioner possessed sole responsibility for his or her patients. Such doctors were literally personal, or family, doctors. They worked alone and had complete autonomy. More recently, district nurses, treatment room nurses, health visitors, social workers, and marriage guidance counsellors, amongst others, have usurped certain aspects of the doctor's role. They have been altering the nature of general practice as, literally, 'personal doctoring', and thus altering the nature of the doctor's independence. Doctors' fears for their independence and autonomy have been exacerbated by the current debate over who, if anyone, should lead the primary health care team. Nurses, health visitors, and social workers are questioning the general practitioner's leadership. The general practitioner has no secure role at the apex of a hierarchy of staff as does the hospital consultant. Consequently, there may be little incentive for doctors adhering to narrow conceptions of their independence to change. As general practitioners have experienced a long history of role and status uncertainty they are likely to be particularly reluctant to yield part of their role to non-physicians. This uncertainty may explain the contradictory attitudes found in some doctors, who complained of lack of time and the amount of trivia they saw but who were still reluctant to delegate extensively, or even at all. For example, one young Welsh doctor, practising from a four-man practice in large purpose-built premises with a treatment room and employed nurse, said:

> 'I'm a bit schizophrenic here I know. On the one hand I would like more time but on the other I don't like the sound of anyone else screening out

all the trivia. Here a consultation fee would be the answer. It would be a means of seeing less and less patients and enabling one to spend more time with the ones that do come.'

General practice is just beginning to recover from the crisis of the mid-1960s. As has previously been pointed out, attempts are currently being made to upgrade general practice. The importance of the general practitioner as a personal, family, and community doctor is continually being stressed. The concept of personal doctoring is dependent on the existence of a good doctor–patient relationship. The expressed fear of losing the patient, or of becoming more distant from the patient, if delegation was practised more extensively may be a fear of losing one of the central features of general practice. Innovations perceived as threatening the doctor–patient relationship and hence the role of the general practitioner are thus resisted.

The doctor–patient relationship was also seen as a symbol of the doctor's independence. This relationship traditionally symbolizes the doctor's freedom from dependence on ancillaries. The relationship with the patient is a personal one, no one comes between doctor and patient. The presence of ancillaries may be seen as threatening this relationship, or depersonalizing it. Thus, doctors adhering to narrow conceptions of independence, namely older doctors, may cling to this relationship to protect it. As the contradictory attitudes discussed suggest, it is not always devotion to the doctor–patient relationship itself which may hinder the development of team care and the practice of delegation, but rather the traditional concepts of clinical and professional freedom.

Although attitudes may change towards the delegation of clinical tasks with an increase in the number of recent graduates entering general practice, doctors with less traditional conceptions of their work, there is no evidence that attitudes may change over the delegation of initial screening in the surgery. Most doctors, whatever their personal characteristics, were hostile towards this concept. Apart from trivia, all that was found was a relationship between favourable attitudes in this area and the practice of a high degree of delegation already. Possibly, as doctors gradually practise a greater amount of clinical delegation in the future, then they will become more receptive towards the concept of the delegation of diagnostic procedures. However, it is doubtful if this will occur on a wide scale unless doctors feel they have a clearly defined role, firmly based on a body of knowledge, and unless they feel their status and autonomy is secure. At present, one of the few clearly defined aspects of the general practitioner's role is that of professional of first contact. Until their role definition goes beyond such superficial descriptions it is unlikely that they will wish to delegate this part of it. In support of this conclusion, a Canadian survey of physicians showed that 93 per cent of physicians wanted to remain the person of first contact, if only to co-ordinate the referral (Warner 1977). Such decision making may also be regarded as part of the autonomy of the profession.

Autonomy is the basis of professionalism and consequently it is not surprising that the medical profession is anxious to preserve it. The suggestion that someone other than the physician sees patients first introduces an element of dependence on assistants which may be seen as anathema to that autonomy. On the other hand, more doctors were willing to relinquish their role of first contact in the home. This aspect of their role seemed to be particularly unpopular and was seen as unnecessarily time consuming. Dajda (1980) found that a large number of prescriptions are written by nurses and receptionists. In the light of this it appears that doctors do not object to the delegation of tasks clearly within their role, as long as the delegation is anonymous and remains unattributable to other named groups. In summary, the medical profession, in theory, clearly wishes to retain its position of autonomy. Interest group politics are a prime force in the resistance of organizations to change. The question which must be answered is whether we can afford a health service based on the private whims of certain doctors.

9

THE INTERVIEWS WITH NURSES

The doctors interviewed were asked if they would agree to the author contacting the community (district) nursing sisters attached to their practices, and also the treatment room nurses who were either employed by them or, in the case of health centres, attached to their practices. These were all state registered nurses. Using this sampling method, doctors' and nurses' statements could be compared. This provided a useful validity check on the procedures delegated in those practices with nursing staff. The comparison of doctors' and nurses' attitudes towards delegation within practices was also of interest.

As has been previously pointed out, district nurses are nurses employed by the area health authority and usually attached to general practitioners' surgeries. A small minority still organize their work on a geographical basis. Their primary function is to provide nursing care in the home; although a number also spend some of their time performing treatments in the surgery. Treatment room nurses are usually employed by the general practitioner, the exception being the case of health centres, where the area health authority is usually the employing body. The main function of treatment room nurses, or practice nurses as they are often known, is to perform treatments in the surgery. Only rarely do they make home visits. They generally undertake delegated medical as well as nursing tasks.

Every doctor with a nurse gave permission for the nurses to be contacted. Area health authorities were then approached for their permission to interview the attached nurses in their employment. Again, this permission was given by all four authorities contacted. Two of these area health authorities provided the author with office space in which to carry out the interviews, and the remaining two gave the author the home telephone numbers of their nurses. One of the authorities even contacted the nurses on the author's behalf. In all, seventy-six nurses were contacted. These consisted of forty-six district nurses and thirty treatment room nurses; five of the latter were attached to health centres by the area health authority. All the nurses agreed to be interviewed, although one district nurse was not seen due to ill health. This resulted in a response rate of 99 per cent.

The interviews

The interviews were carried out either in the nurses' own homes, in the doctors' practices, or in the accommodation provided by the area health authorities. They were conducted between May and September 1977. Most interviews lasted between one and two hours and, as with the doctors' interviews, they were semi-structured. They were designed to obtain quantitative data about procedures performed, and also to obtain qualitative information about nurses' attitudes towards performing delegated medical tasks. The same statistical techniques that were used to analyse the doctors' results were used to analyse nurses' results. Finally, it should be pointed out that where doctors employed, or had attached, more than one treatment room nurse, each nurse was interviewed.

The nurse working in the surgery

'I'm a district nurse, not a practice nurse. I don't want to spend my time in the surgery, I'd miss out on the community work.'
(District nurse in Wales)

All nurses were asked how much time they spent performing treatments in the surgery. As would be expected, the treatment room nurses spent longest in the surgery. Forty-seven per cent of the treatment room nurses worked eight to ten surgery sessions per week, in contrast to 2 per cent of the district nurses. Fifty-three per cent of treatment room nurses worked five to seven surgery sessions per week in contrast to 4 per cent of district nurses. Twenty-seven per cent of district nurses worked one hour or less in the surgery five times a week, and 27 per cent worked an hour or less in the surgery less than five times a week. Forty per cent of district nurses did not perform treatments in the surgery at all. The limited periods spent by district nurses in the surgery may be explained by the fact that home nursing is their primary function, and they may lack both the time and the inclination to perform more treatments in the surgery.

Treatment room work does not necessarily include the performance of delegated medical duties. District nurses, for example, often
perform nursing treatments, such as dressings, in the surgery for their
own patients who have recovered sufficiently to travel. This saves the
nurse's own travelling time. As one district nurse in Wales said:

> 'Doing these things, injections, dressings, in the surgery saves my own
> time as my patients who can walk come to the surgery to see me. This
> saves my own time which would otherwise be spent travelling around
> to do the same procedures in people's homes.'

When a treatment room nurse is employed by, or attached to, a
practice then the district nurse may refer all newly mobile patients
who require treatment to that nurse. This does lead to a certain
amount of role overlap and good communications are essential if
conflict is to be minimized. This potential danger was pointed out by
a young district nurse in Wales who was attached to a large group
practice with an employed treatment room nurse:

> 'If my patients can get to the surgery then I encourage them to do so and
> the practice nurse treats them. I don't do anything in the surgery at all.
> I know some nurses feel resentful when the doctor suddenly employs
> his own nurse and so the nurses sometimes lose their patients, but Dr X
> has always had a practice nurse so I've never felt pushed out. We have
> a very good relationship. I don't feel she invades my territory at all.'

Alternatively, these two types of nurse sometimes work together performing surgery treatments. Another district nurse in Wales, again
attached to a large group practice with an employed treatment room
nurse, stated that there were no role boundaries between the nurses in
the surgery:

> 'I occasionally work in the surgery even though there are two practice
> nurses. We all lend a hand with each other's work. I think all the fuss
> about demarcations and boundaries is ridiculous. If I have any spare
> time I go back to the surgery and lend a hand with whatever's going on.'

Thus, while in some practices there are clear role divisions between
district and treatment room nurses, in others these divisions are
blurred. Do differences exist in the type of work performed in the
surgery by these two types of nurses?

Delegated procedures performed by nurses in the surgery

'I'm lucky, Dr Y does his own work. He doesn't delegate anything.
Nursing is nursing, and the doctor's work is his own.'

(District nurse in Surrey)

Which procedures are performed by both types of nurse and with what frequency? Nurses were shown a list of clinical, technical, and diagnostic procedures of varying complexity and asked whether, and how often, they performed them. The list of procedures nurses were asked about was more comprehensive than that shown to doctors. *Table 3* indicates the total number of nurses performing clinical procedures in the surgery and the frequency with which they were performed. *Table 4* shows this breakdown by type of nurse.

Table 3   *Proportion of nurses performing clinical tasks in the surgery*

| | Proportion of nurses performing task: | | | Total |
	regularly	occasionally	never	
injections, dressings, suture removal	33%	36%	31%	
immunizations and vaccinations	23%	21%	56%	
ear syringing	37%	25%	38%	
venepuncture	15%	17%	68%	75
cervical cytology	6%	3%	91%	
minor surgical tasks such as incision of boils	—	5%	95%	

Source: Bowling, A. (1980) 'To do or not to do'. *Nursing Mirror*, July 17: 31.
Reprinted with permission.

Injections, dressings and suture removal and ear syringing were the tasks performed most frequently in the surgery. As *Table 4* shows, marked differences were evident in the regularity with which tasks were performed by district nurses in comparison with treatment room (practice) nurses.

Nurses who performed three to five of the listed clinical tasks in *Tables 3* and *4* on a regular basis were classified as performing a high number of delegated tasks in the surgery. Those who performed less than this on a regular or occasional basis, or who performed at least three tasks but only occasionally, were classified as performing a low number of delegated tasks. A third category was created for those performing none of the listed tasks at all in the surgery.

Twenty-nine per cent of the nurses performed a high number of tasks by this classification, 47 per cent performed a low number, and 24 per cent performed none of the tasks in the surgery. All those in the

Table 4   *Type of nurse performing clinical tasks in the surgery*

	Proportion of practice nurses performing task:			Number of nurses
	regularly	occasionally	never	
injections, dressings, suture removal	80%	20%	—	⎫
immunizations and vaccinations	57%	43%	—	⎬ 30
ear syringing	80%	17%	3%	
venepuncture	37%	23%	40%	
cervical cytology	17%	7%	76%	
minor surgical tasks	—	13%	87%	⎭

	Proportion of district nurses performing task:			
injections, dressings, suture removal	2%	49%	49%	⎫
immunizations and vaccinations	—	16%	84%	⎬
ear syringing	9%	31%	60%	⎬ 45
venepuncture	—	13%	87%	
cervical cytology	—	—	100%	
minor surgical tasks	—	—	100%	⎭

last group were district nurses, as were 77 per cent of those performing a low number of tasks. In contrast, all those who performed three or more of the tasks regularly were treatment room nurses. In addition and as would be expected from the interviews with the doctors, most nurses performing a high number of tasks worked in practices containing three or more doctors, 91 per cent, in comparison with 57 per cent of those performing a low number and 61 per cent of those performing none.

Again, as may be expected, treatment room nurses were more likely to say they had access to treatment rooms, 80 per cent in comparison with 48 per cent of the district nurses. Where these were not available, either the reception area or a spare consulting room was used for treatments. Access to an adequately equipped treatment room area would undoubtedly facilitate the delegation of tasks.

As *Tables 5* and *6* show, nurses performed the various technical procedures in the surgery even less often than the clinical tasks listed. Once again treatment room nurses were more likely to perform these procedures than district nurses.

Table 5   *Proportion of nurses performing technical tasks in the surgery*

	Proportion of nurses performing task:			Total
	regularly	occasionally	never	
blood pressure recording	20%	21%	59%	
electrocardiogram recording (ECG)	12%	3%	85%	
erythrocyte sediment-ation rate estimation (ESR)	5%	—	95%	75
haemoglobin level estimation (HB)	9%	—	91%	

Source: Bowling, A. (1980) 'To do or not to do'. *Nursing Mirror*, July 17: 31.
Reprinted with permission.

Table 6   *Type of nurse performing technical tasks in the surgery*

	Proportion of practice nurses performing task:			Number of nurses
	regularly	occasionally	never	
blood pressure recording	50%	30%	20%	
electrocardiogram recording (ECG)	27%	—	73%	
erythrocyte sediment-ation rate estimation (ESR)	10%	—	90%	30
haemoglobin level estimation (HB)	17%	—	83%	
	Proportion of district nurses performing task:			
blood pressure recording	—	16%	84%	
electrocardiogram recording (ECG)	2%	4%	94%	
erythrocyte sediment-ation rate estimation (ESR)	2%	—	98%	45
haemoglobin level estimation (HB)	4%	—	96%	

As doctors did not usually perform ECGs, ESR, or HB, it appears that patients requiring these procedures generally have to be referred to hospital. In the case of ESR and HB the patient's blood may have been taken in the surgery and the sample sent to the hospital pathology laboratory. However, as the majority of doctors did not delegate venepuncture it appears that whichever method was utilized neither was very efficient.

Attitudes towards performing delegated clinical and technical tasks

'Delegation is really getting away from nursing.'

(District nurse in Surrey)

Overall, nurses were no more in favour of performing delegated clinical tasks than doctors were of delegating them. The number of nurses not performing particular tasks regularly, but who were in favour of doing so, rarely exceeded two-thirds and was sometimes considerably lower. For example, of those nurses not regularly performing injections, dressings, and suture removal in the surgery, 70 per cent were in favour of doing so. Of those not regularly performing immunizations and vaccinations in the surgery 67 per cent were in favour of doing these tasks. Fifty-seven per cent of those not regularly performing ear syringing held favourable attitudes on this issue, as did 61 per cent of those not regularly performing vene-puncture. Fifty-four per cent of nurses not performing cervical cytology regularly were in favour of doing this, and 55 per cent were in favour of performing minor surgical procedures. The range of proportions of nurses in favour of doing particular tasks was similar on the issue of technical procedures. For example, 75 per cent of nurses not regularly taking blood pressure in the surgery were in favour of doing so, 45 per cent of those not regularly taking ECGs were in favour of doing them; 51 per cent of those not estimating ESR and 48 per cent of those not regularly estimating HB held favourable attitudes towards performing them. However, taking those nurses who did not perform any one particular delegated clinical or technical procedure regularly in the surgery, in no instance would more than 41 per cent have been willing to actually perform them themselves. Again, in view of the relatively simple nature of these tasks, these figures are, on the whole, disappointing.

Nurses were divided into two groups. The first group consisted of those nurses who were in favour of nurses performing no fewer than four of the six listed clinical tasks. These were classified as nurses with favourable attitudes towards performing delegated clinical tasks. The second group included those in favour of performing three or fewer of the tasks and those not in favour of performing any. These were classified as the group with unfavourable attitudes. Sixty-seven per cent of nurses were included in the first group and 33 per cent in the second. These groupings were similar to the equivalent groupings for doctors, where the proportions concerning favourability to delegation were 63 per cent and 37 per cent respectively.

A similar classification was used with nurses concerning attitudes towards performing technical tasks in the surgery. The first group included those nurses in favour of nurses performing at least three of the four listed tasks; this was classified as the group with favourable attitudes. All other nurses were categorized as having unfavourable attitudes towards performing technical tasks. Fifty-three per cent of nurses were included in the first group and 47 per cent in the second.

Nurses with favourable attitudes towards performing both types of tasks were more likely to be treatment room nurses. For example, 58 per cent of treatment room nurses favoured the performance of clinical tasks, in comparison with 4 per cent of the district nurses; and 60 per cent favoured the performance of technical procedures, in comparison with 17 per cent of district nurses. It appears that the prospects for expanding the role of the treatment room nurse in the surgery are more encouraging than the prospects for expanding the role of the district nurse in this area. Given the choice, district nurses prefer to retain their central role of giving nursing care in the patient's home, rather than combining this to a greater extent with performing delegated tasks in the surgery.

Reasons given by nurses for their attitudes towards delegation

'You have to advance with the world. It's nice to be part of it rather than be left behind.'

(District nurse in Surrey)

When asked an open question on their views on performing delegated medical tasks, nurses mentioned six advantages and seven disadvantages. Some of these were mutually exclusive. For example, 70 per cent said that performing delegated medical tasks increases the level of satisfaction nurses derive from their work. One young Welsh district nurse said:

'I would like to do more, it makes nursing more interesting. If you have the right equipment and the right surgery there's no reason why nurses could not do more in the surgery. I assisted the doctor to remove a lump from a woman's bottom once. There's no reason why it shouldn't become a more regular part of my work. It's more interesting than just doing dull routine things.'

Such comments indicate that many nurses currently find their nursing roles routine and boring. Taking on more medical tasks may stimulate more interest and thus increase nurses' satisfaction with their work. On the other hand, 21 per cent of nurses argued strongly that expanded roles in the surgery would be less satisfying. One of the district nurses expressing this view said:

> 'My day is spent washing people, the doctors I'm attached to prefer to do everything else themselves. I was trained to bath people. That's what a nurse is for, otherwise how would I build up a relationship with people?'

However, the majority of nurses did not hold this view. Nurses often chose their occupation because they wanted to give practical help and care to patients. Performing delegated medical tasks, such as taking blood, may conform with this aim. It also conforms with the common stereotype of the nurse as the doctor's assistant. It is usually only when nurses become aware of the issue of professionalization, and when they are promoted to higher levels, that their role is perceived differently. At that point it is no longer seen in terms of assisting doctors, nor necessarily always in terms of helping patients, but is viewed in terms of what is best for nursing as a profession. Unfortunately, what is regarded as best for nursing as a profession is not necessarily best for nurses themselves in terms of personal satisfaction through their work. The movement of nurses away from patient care and towards administrative and managerial functions is one example of this process.

Whatever the implications of delegation for nurses' satisfaction with their work, the fact remains that nursing is currently attempting to establish its own professional identity. It is not considered professional to undertake tasks belonging to another professional group because one criterion of professionalism is the development of a unique body of knowledge, which is related to the crucial issue of autonomy of action. Thus, as nursing is attempting to establish its independence from the medical profession, nursing leaders are resisting many of the attempts by doctors to delegate medical tasks to nurses. The issue of professional status was mentioned by only a minority of nurses in this study. For example, while 8 per cent felt that performing delegated medical tasks enhances the status of nursing, a further 15 per cent said that it lowers the status of the profession. These conflicting views can be clearly seen in the following statements, both made by district nurses in Wales:

> 'I would like to do all these things listed as the more we are able to do the more the status of the profession increases.'

> 'Delegation may save the doctor's time but by implication the nurse's time is seen as less valuable. I think all this business of delegation is really pure pig-headedness on the part of the doctor, with only his time being saved. There's no way we are going to be treated as equal health professionals with that attitude.'

It is possible that so few nurses mentioned the issue of professional status because it remains a preoccupation of nursing leaders and academics. More nurses, however, were conscious of the related debate on the role of the nurse. For example, 51 per cent argued that the performance of delegated medical tasks is not within the scope of the nurse's role. Eighty-four per cent of these nurses were district nurses. It is perhaps surprising that 16 per cent were treatment room nurses. The chosen role of these nurses is generally to assist the doctor. In contrast, the main function of the district nurse is to provide care in patients' homes. Despite the fact that district nurses now spend more time in the surgery than at any other period of their history, they still see their role, on the whole, as quite distinct from that of treatment room nurses. The caring image of the nurse predominates in their minds, as can be seen from the following two statements. Both were made by district nurses in Wales, neither of whom performed any delegated medical tasks in the surgery:

> 'I prefer nursing as it used to be. It was more like caring in the past. It's too technical now. It would become even more technical with more delegation.'

> 'In hospital nurses are too Americanized. To me it isn't nursing any more. That's why I decided to do district nursing, you still care for the patient as a district nurse. Sometimes patients come home to an empty house so we have to boil the kettle for them, look for some clean clothes, light the fire. If I didn't go in I don't know how patients would manage. If you're in the community it really is nursing. Nurses in hospital, just like those who work in the surgery, are just like technicians. They're getting away from nursing.'

However, one young treatment room nurse, working in a group practice in Wales, pointed out that whether or not tasks can be strictly defined as nursing tasks often depends on the way they are approached:

> 'In the strict hospital sense our work isn't nursing. But it all depends on how you treat people and how you get to know them. You find it means a lot to remember something a patient has told you on a previous occasion and ask them about that particular thing next time you see them, particularly with the elderly who often have no one to remember them. To me that is nursing.'

This argument is similar to those put forward by members of the nursing profession in the United States and Canada in their attempts to point to the distinctions between the role of the physician's assistant and that of the nurse practitioner. The latter contributes caring to the more technical role. The addition of caring to an essentially technical task was clearly described by a district nurse in Surrey who felt strongly that nurses should not act as the doctor's assistant:

'We should be devoting more time to supportive work rather than taking on the doctor's work. What was it Charlotte Kratz said? "You can teach a monkey to give an injection but you can't teach a monkey to do what you're doing while you're giving the injection." Talking is so important.'

Ironically, this statement could also be used to support the argument for an expanded nursing role in the surgery. It is the addition of the caring element to the role which would allow nurses to retain their identity.

However, not all nurses arguing that delegated medical tasks are not within the role of the nurse saw nursing in terms of its traditional bedside caring function. Thirteen per cent of these nurses referred to the current attempts to professionalize nursing by developing the role of the clinical nurse specialist and other nurse specialist or consultancy roles. For example, one district nurse in Surrey said:

'Before nurses start doing the doctor's work there's a lot of work in our own field we should be looking at. The clinical nurse specialist is a field we could work in. That's a specialist's job which involves knowing what's available when people consult you.'

That there is some disagreement among nurses over their role definition is further seen in the final example of a district nurse, also from Surrey, who was willing to take on as much as possible of the doctor's work:

'The role of the nurse is changing tremendously and if you are only going to perform what you regard as traditional nursing duties – bathing, injections, dressings and so on – then you are going to get left behind. At one time I used to do all the bathing, but now I have a nursing auxiliary to do it all. You don't need a nurse's training to give baths.'

Nursing, like general practice, is undergoing its own identity crisis. This crisis is reflected not only in the literature and in official reports on nurses, but also in nurses' attitudes themselves. In view of this, it is not unexpected that many nurses were reluctant to undertake delegated medical tasks, tasks which legitimately belong to another professional group. However, as treatment room nurses were less likely to argue that medical tasks are not within their role there is certainly future potential for an expanded surgery role for these nurses for they have already chosen a role which includes the performance of medical tasks. Moreover, as they often seemed to enter general practice settings because of the flexibility of the working hours, which fitted in with their family commitments, it is possible that there will always be a ready supply of such nurses. For example, one treatment room nurse, working in a large health centre in Wales, said:

> 'This sort of work is no good if you want a career. There's no pro-motion prospects or anything. It's no good for a single girl. I only do this because I'm married and I have children to look after. It's so difficult to get part-time work in hospitals now.'

Other treatment room nurses often made similar remarks about their work. They would refer to themselves as 'doctors' skivvies', and as 'general all-rounders – washer up, cleaner . . .'. One treatment room nurse even referred to her job as 'slavery'. These reports tend to confirm the fears of nurses who believe that delegation would lower the status of nursing. Perhaps there would be less discontent if the role of the treatment room nurse was more systematically organized, and if official recognition was given to the work of these nurses by the organization of mandatory, national training courses. The uniform employment of treatment room nurses by health authorities, rather than doctors, may remove some of the feelings of isolation. It would also have the additional advantage of making them professionally responsible to other nurses. As one treatment room nurse in a three-man practice in Surrey said:

> 'The main problem of working as a practice nurse is that you're divorced from the NHS. You're a privately employed nurse. We would like to be part of a recognized body of nurses. If doctors are going to delegate more and more to us we should have a recognized status.'

Four other advantages of undertaking delegated medical tasks were mentioned by nurses. Thirty-four per cent said that the advantage was the saving of the doctor's time. Sixty-two per cent of the treatment room nurses felt this in comparison with 38 per cent of the district nurses. Treatment room nurses are likely to be aware that one of the functions of their employment is to save the doctor's time by a more efficient distribution of skills. Seventeen per cent of nurses also said that delegation saves the patient's waiting time, 8 per cent said that it results in a better distribution of skills, and 8 per cent said that it enhances the nurse–doctor relationship. Nurses mentioning the last advantage felt that doctors showed more respect for them if they could perform medical tasks. Again, this goes against the current attempts to establish an independent professional identity for nurses. One of these nurses, who was a district nurse but who also performed treatments in the surgery, said:

> 'To work in the surgery and perform delegated tasks enables you to have much closer contact with the doctors. You really feel you're a member of the team rather than being an underdog as in the past. Doctors used to look at us as if all we knew was how to bath a patient.'

Four other problems with, or disadvantages of, delegation were mentioned. For example, 19 per cent of nurses said they would not want the greater responsibility involved in performing delegated medical tasks. These nurses were more likely to be district nurses than treatment room nurses, 79 per cent in comparison with 56 per cent. Also, 21 per cent of nurses said they were insufficiently trained to undertake any medical tasks. Few of the nurses interviewed had received formal instruction, whilst training or from the area health authority, in the performance of tasks such as venepuncture or ear syringing. Most had relied on instruction from the doctors they worked with if such tasks were undertaken. The haphazard nature of such instruction was described by several nurses. For example, one treatment room nurse in a large group practice in Wales said:

> 'When I first trained, the matron in hospital wouldn't allow nurses to take blood. So when I came here and the doctor asked me to take blood I was a bit nervous. I agreed to do it when he said he'd come in and watch me do the first few. But when it came to it he only stayed for two and then said "That's fine, just carry on".'

Nurses who performed delegated tasks and those in favour of performing these tasks were asked if they felt a national training course in treatment room work needed to be set up. The majority, 95 per cent, said 'yes'.

Twenty-four per cent of the nurses interviewed stated that one main problem which would have to be overcome before delegation could become more widespread is doctor opposition. Most of these nurses were treatment room nurses, 58 per cent in comparison with 34 per cent of district nurses. As these nurses have more contact with doctors they may be more conscious of their prejudices in this area. One Welsh treatment room nurse, who did more receptionist work than nursing, complained bitterly about doctors' reluctance to delegate more tasks to her:

> 'They think they're little tin gods, they don't want to give away any of their power.'

Some of these nurses reported feelings of frustration because the doctors they worked with would perform procedures they themselves had been taught to perform. For example, one treatment room nurse, again in Wales, said the doctor would even do dressings himself:

> 'Dr X does all the dressings himself, he enjoys it. He comes in here (treatment room) and does it. He'll spend half an hour doing a wart with a whole queue of patients waiting. He'll do it even with me sitting here doing nothing. I say to him "Let me do it", but he won't. He says he likes to do it himself. But then he moans about work piling up.'

One district nurse who performed treatments such as dressings in the surgery complained about interference from the doctor:

> 'Dr Y is a very old-fashioned doctor. She likes to check everything I do. She even has to see if the dressings I do are OK. She has to decide herself which dressings I use.'

It appears that many doctors employed their own nurses partly for receptionist duties, including answering the telephone, rather than for the performance of a wide range of delegated duties. Several nurses felt that doctors underestimated their nursing and technical skills. As one of the district nurses said:

> 'The type of work you do often depends on the GP and what he thinks you're capable of doing. GPs should be better educated over what nurses are capable of doing. Too often they think nurses are only capable of first-aid and bathing, especially those doctors over fifty.'

Finally, 8 per cent of nurses expressed anxieties over their legal position in the event of a mishap while performing delegated medical tasks. Some confusion generally existed among nurses regarding their legal position. Nurses performing delegated procedures were asked a direct question about this. Eighty-two per cent of them believed the doctor took complete responsibility for their actions. These tended to be treatment room nurses, 91 per cent in comparison with 60 per cent of district nurses. All those who felt the doctor would not take responsibility for their actions were members of the Royal College of Nursing. In contrast, only 54 per cent of those who believed doctors would take responsibility were members. Moreover, 27 per cent of nurses believing that the doctor would take responsibility for their actions were not legally protected by virtue of College membership or membership of a trade union. Altogether, 64 per cent of nurses in the sample were members of a professional nursing body, such as the Royal College of Nursing or, in the case of some of those who also had a midwifery qualification, the Royal College of Midwives. Seventeen per cent were members of a trade union and 19 per cent belonged to neither. This last group showed no intention of joining either type of organization. For example, one treatment room nurse who worked in a large health centre in Wales said:

'I don't belong to the RCN or a trade union. Dr X said he'd stick up for me if anything happens. It's so expensive to belong . . . . It's so much money to pay out yearly just on the offchance that something may happen.'

District nurses were more likely than treatment room nurses to have taken out legal coverage for themselves, 96 per cent in comparison with 60 per cent. Perhaps these nurses are more likely to be encouraged to do so by the health authorities who employ them. In such circumstances it is difficult to see how nurses can safely be encouraged to expand their role. Treatment room nurses often appeared to believe that their work included little responsibility. One such nurse employed by two doctors in Surrey said:

'I would do all these listed things. The responsibility wouldn't worry me a scrap, the doctor covers me. That's why I'm happy being a practice nurse, there's no personal responsibility. I don't want any responsibility.'

Not only does the limited membership of professional bodies among nurses question the status of nursing as a profession, but nurses' deference to doctors and their lack of desire for responsibility detracts from any image nursing may have of itself as a profession equal to and independent of medicine. This deference can be seen in the following statement made by a district nurse working in a three-man practice in Surrey:

'If a doctor asks you to do something you do it. They're trying to separate us from doctors now by having their own management. It was better before. I'm pleased to help the doctor.'

Similar statements were made by several of the older district nurses. Other nurses, primarily engaged in district nursing, said they deferred to the doctor's orders in order to maintain a good working relationship. However, they often did so against their own wishes. One district nurse commented: 'It's all very well for the nursing officers to tell us we can't do this and that, but we have to work with the doctors.' Such conflicts may partly explain why 31 per cent of the district nurses said that they would like to see the introduction of structured guidelines on delegation. Few treatment room nurses agreed. District nurses, with their dual responsibilities, sometimes saw guidelines as a solution to their dilemma of whose instructions to obey – the doctor's or those of the area health authority nursing officers. As one of them said: 'If we had guidelines saying what we could and could not do then doctors would not be able to expect us to do things that we are not sure about.'

Nurses not performing particular delegated procedures regularly, but who were in favour of doing so, were asked why they did not do them. Twenty-eight per cent said they had no equipment. For example, one district nurse attached to a four-man practice in Wales said:

> 'If I want to take a blood pressure I have to come in here (doctor's consulting room) to borrow the blood pressure machine. It's really awkward not having one. Then you need an aural spec. when you do the ear syringing. I have to borrow the doctors'. I'm sure they hide it when they think I want to borrow it. I even have to use their syringes for the ear syringing.'

Thirty-one per cent of nurses mentioned lack of space as a constraint. For example, many of the district nurses could perform treatments only when one of the doctors' consulting rooms was available. Other reasons given were: lack of time, 42 per cent; opposition from doctors, 28 per cent; opposition from the area health authority, 9 per cent; 7 per cent, all district nurses, said they would like to work in the surgery but the doctor employed a treatment room nurse.

In reply to a direct question, 73 per cent of nurses said they would like to expand their clinical role in the surgery. Fifty-eight per cent of these, however, felt they were unable to do so because of lack of time. A quarter of the nurses interviewed said they did have time to perform more delegated tasks. However, while 43 per cent of the treatment room nurses felt they had time to undertake further duties, the figure for district nurses was just 13 per cent. District nurses were asked how much of their own work could be delegated to state enrolled nurses and to nursing auxiliaries. Twenty-nine per cent felt that much of their work could be delegated and 60 per cent felt little could be. The argument that the doctor's time could be saved, and a better distribution of skills effected, by delegation to nurses is not logical in a situation in which nurses also have little time. District and treatment room nurses, or treatment room nurses alone, may have to reorganize their workloads in the future to enable them to undertake an expanded surgery role. They too, may have to practise more delegation. The alternative is the introduction of other types of personnel to do this work. Whichever course of action is taken depends on the future attitudes of doctors and nurses to delegation. These, in turn, depend on how their roles are defined and the level of their professional status.

The performance of tasks requiring the exercise of autonomy

'We're not diagnosticians, it's not part of our role.'

(District nurse in Wales)

Nurses were also asked about the performance of tasks involving the exercise of autonomy, or independent decision making. These included the supervision of clinics, for example family planning; the initial preparation of patients in the surgery together with brief history taking before the patient sees the doctor; the assessment of patients without appointments to decide on the urgency of their treatment; and the performance of initial home visits for diagnostic purposes. Twenty-four per cent of nurses said they supervised clinics regularly; 57 per cent of treatment room nurses and 2 per cent of district nurses did this. Five per cent of nurses initially prepared patients for the doctor and took medical histories regularly. These were all treatment room nurses working in one practice in Surrey. The practice was highly organized with a series of consulting rooms. Patients would enter one room to be prepared and have a medical history taken and would then wait to see the doctor while the nurses prepared following patients. Thirty-five per cent of nurses assessed patients without appointments, or casual attenders as they are often known, on a regular basis and 4 per cent did this occasionally. Again, these were all treatment room nurses. Sixteen per cent of nurses undertook initial home visiting, but only occasionally. Twenty-two per cent of district nurses made such visits in comparison with 7 per cent of treatment room nurses. Nurses were also asked about the performance of initial screening in the surgery in order to decide if patients needed to see the doctor. As would be expected, no nurse currently undertook this role. This is discussed separately further on. The distinctions between the role of the district nurse and that of the treatment room nurse are quite clear here. Initial home visiting is the main procedure requiring the exercise of autonomy undertaken by district nurses. On the other hand, procedures performed in the surgery requiring the exercise of autonomy are the domain of the treatment room nurse.

Attitudes towards performing delegated tasks requiring autonomy

'I could say to a patient "You don't need to see the doctor" and that patient may die. I wouldn't want the responsibility.'

(Treatment room nurse in Surrey)

What did nurses think of performing procedures requiring the exercise of their judgement? Sixty-two per cent of nurses not regularly preparing patients for the doctor and taking medical histories were in favour of doing so. Fifty-four per cent of nurses not regularly supervising clinics were in favour of doing this, and 55 per cent of those not assessing patients without appointments were also in favour of doing so. Fewer were in favour of undertaking initial home visits – 25 per cent. In each of these cases approximately a fifth to a quarter of nurses would not actually undertake these tasks themselves, despite the expression of favourable views.

Forty-four per cent of nurses were in favour of performing all four of these tasks regularly. These nurses were more likely to be treatment room nurses, 64 per cent, than district nurses, 21 per cent. Nurses already performing these tasks tended to be more confident in their abilities and this often appeared to be due to the existence of support from the doctors. For example, as one district nurse who undertook initial home visiting said:

'I do initial home visiting occasionally. I'm quite happy about doing them because I know that the doctors will come out if I ask them to. I'm quite confident in my ability to assess patients' conditions as I've been on the district a long time, nineteen years, so I'm quite experienced.'

Thus the most popular procedure here was the initial preparation of patients for the doctor, together with brief medical history taking. This requires the exercise of the least amount of autonomy, and hence responsibility. Furthermore, nurses could often see more advantages for the patient in this method of organization. One of the treatment room nurses actually doing this work said:

'The use of a nurse to prepare patients for the doctor ensures that patients are examined properly. Lots of doctors just slip the stethoscope under your blouse. They don't ask the patient to undress. When the nurse prepares the patient the doctor is bound to listen to the patient's chest and back.'

Related to the issue of autonomy are the findings that a minority of nurses performed certain procedures for patients without the patient first having to see the doctor. Of those who undertook ear syringing, 21 per cent performed it on their own initiative. These nurses made it known to patients that this was their function and so patients tended to consult them directly over blocked ears. Thirty-two per cent of those doing immunizations and vaccinations performed them without the patient first seeing the doctor. Finally, 41 per cent of nurses said they provided simple emergency care, such as the dressing and cleansing of wounds and administering tetanus injections. Twenty-six per cent of these nurses provided this service without the patient necessarily seeing the doctor first. These practices suggest a need to recognize and systematically organize the delegation of medical tasks to nurses, otherwise the present confusion over legal responsibilities and roles will continue.

What about nurses' attitudes towards the initial screening of patients in the surgery to decide who needs to see the doctor and who can be treated without a consultation? Thirty-nine per cent of nurses were in favour of a nurse undertaking this task and, of these, 28 per cent even felt that nurses needed no further preparation for this role. A further 7 per cent were in favour of a specially trained assistant undertaking such screening, and not a nurse. Altogether, then, 45 per cent of all nurses were in favour of a non-physician initially screening patients in the surgery, in contrast to just 27 per cent of the doctors. While doctors appeared reluctant to relinquish their position of professional of first contact in the surgery, but were more enthusiastic over delegating initial home visits, the reverse was found to be true among nurses. They preferred to undertake a screening role in the surgery rather than in the home. This was usually because they felt this required less responsibility. For example, one district nurse in Surrey commented:

'I wouldn't mind seeing patients first in the surgery, but I wouldn't do it in the home. In the surgery there's always the doctor there if you need any advice, but he's not there in the home.'

Nurses in favour of initial screening in the surgery were more likely to have qualified in or after 1960, 68 per cent in comparison with 49 per cent of other nurses; and they were also more likely to be in favour of performing all four of the previously mentioned autonomous tasks, 53 per cent in contrast to 37 per cent of nurses not in favour. It is perhaps surprising that no significant differences emerged between district and treatment room nurses on this issue. However, although 39 per

cent were in favour of nurses performing initial screening, 31 per cent
of these nurses would not have been willing to undertake this task
themselves.

When questioned openly about the advantages they saw in such a
scheme, 29 per cent of nurses saw these mainly from the doctors' point
of view. These nurses said initial screening would save the doctors'
time. They tended to hold strong views on the amount of time wasted
by trivial consultations. For example, one treatment room nurse in a
purpose-built practice in Wales said:

> 'A lot of patients come unnecessarily to me, but then a lot come unneces-
> sarily to the doctor. They've got a headache but won't give themselves
> an aspirin. At least 50 per cent of those who come don't need to see
> the doctor. An assistant in the supermarket dropped a can of beans on
> her foot a few weeks ago and conked out. They brought her in here. If
> we weren't here they wouldn't have bothered. A bucket of cold water
> over her head was all she needed.'

Fewer nurses mentioned the advantages of initial screening in the
surgery from the point of view of the nurse. Ironically, those who did
were all treatment room nurses: nurses who have chosen to assist the
doctor. For example, 20 per cent of nurses said that if they undertook
initial screening they would derive more satisfaction from their work,
and five per cent said that such a role would enhance the status of
nursing. Of course, such replies would be less likely from district
nurses as they have elected to give nursing care mainly in patients'
homes in a more traditional fashion.

Far more disadvantages of such a method of organization were
mentioned. In general, although the arguments presented were
similar to those forwarded on the issue of the performance of
delegated clinical tasks, the proportions raising each issue were
smaller. In contrast, doctors' prejudices and fears emerged more
strongly on the subject of initial screening. Just 32 per cent of the
nurses said that the performance of initial screening is not within their
role. Seventy per cent of these nurses qualified before 1960 in contrast
to 31 per cent of nurses not raising this issue. These nurses also tended
to emphasize the caring, rather than the technical, aspects of their
role: 'This is getting away from nursing, I wouldn't want to be a mini-
doctor'; 'We're not diagnosticians, it's not part of our role.' A number
of these nurses also expressed concern about the effect such a role
would have on the professional status of nursing. They felt that nurses
should concentrate on their own role rather than take over part of that
belonging to another profession.

Thirty-two per cent of nurses felt that only fully qualified doctors could safely diagnose. In contrast, 51 per cent of doctors had presented this argument. This difference is to be expected as doctors would be experiencing direct role threat from another professional group. However, it appears that nurses, as well as doctors, and even patients, need re-educating before such a system could be introduced. They tended to feel that, as one nurse said: 'It's dangerous to have someone who's undertrained.'

More nurses than doctors said that patient acceptance of such a system would never be achieved, 37 per cent in comparison with 28 per cent. They believed that this implied that such a method of practice could not be implemented. As two treatment room nurses in Surrey said:

'I think there would be a punch-up out there in the waiting room if any-one said they weren't ill enough to see the doctor.'

'Do you honestly think the British public, when they can get treatment free, would accept a second-class opinion? This would all depend on educating the public and you cannot change people's attitudes over-night. Even now they're only just coming round to accepting group practices. Patients still get very discontented when they cannot even see the doctor of their choice.'

Fewer nurses, 20 per cent, felt that doctor opposition to initial screening would prevent the concept being implemented in practice. These nurses realized that doctors would feel professionally threat-ened by such a scheme: 'They would feel their province is being threatened.' Five per cent of nurses even maintained that doctors could become obsolete with such a system in operation. Two Welsh district nurses commented: 'If nurses were trained to diagnose we wouldn't need doctors', 'I could see the doctor sitting there all day waiting for patients to be referred.'

Other disadvantages were mentioned by smaller numbers of nurses. For example, 9 per cent said they personally would not want the extra responsibility incurred in a screening role; 8 per cent felt that screening by a non-physician would interfere with the doctor–patient relationship; 7 per cent argued that the legal complications would be too great; and 5 per cent even said there was no need for initial screening as, to quote one district nurse in Wales: 'Doctors are not so overworked as to warrant such a change'.

In contrast to doctors, then, nurses' views on disadvantages did not emerge more strongly on the issue of screening than on the issue of the delegation of clinical tasks. On the other hand, when asked directly whether or not they were in favour of such a system and, if so, whether they would undertake such a role, nurses' attitudes were far less favourable, although, again, they were more favourable than doctors'. Such a finding is not necessarily surprising as this issue presents nurses with less of a role and professional threat than doctors. On the other hand, the function and status of the nurse would be faced with uncertainty if the tasks of another professional group were performed, particularly in the case of nurses undertaking more complex diagnostic work.

Summary and discussion

The proportion of nurses performing delegated clinical, technical, or autonomous procedures on a regular basis were low, although they were higher among treatment room nurses with the exception of initial home visiting. Forty per cent of the treatment room nurses never performed a relatively uncomplicated task such as venepuncture, a procedure delegated to either technicians or nurses in hospitals. Similarly, only 50 per cent of these nurses recorded blood pressures, again a procedure which could easily be delegated.

Overall, nurses appeared no more in favour of performing the clinical tasks listed than doctors were of delegating them. The number of nurses not performing a particular task, but in favour of doing so, rarely exceeded two-thirds; and was often far lower, despite the simple nature of most of the tasks in question. Treatment room nurses were far more likely to hold favourable attitudes towards undertaking the listed procedures. On the other hand, a significant minority of these still had reservations.

Nurses, as well as doctors, found the concept of initial screening by a non-physician to be controversial. However, while doctors were less in favour of a non-physician acting as an initial contact in the surgery, they were more in favour of delegating this role in the home. On the other hand, nurses appeared more nervous about undertaking a screening role in the home than in the surgery, for the most part because they felt the responsibility was greater in the home. Nurses evidently feel less role threat over the concept of initial surgery screening than doctors, despite the implications the operation of such a scheme would have for the role and professional status of the nurse. In fact, 45 per cent of the nurses were in favour of this scheme, although not all of these would have been willing to undertake initial screening themselves.

Although the prospects for expanding the role of the treatment room nurse appear more optimistic than those for the community nurse, on the whole nurses still seemed uncertain and confused about the advisability of performing medical tasks. For example, 70 per cent of the nurses said that performing delegated medical tasks increases nurses' level of work satisfaction, and 73 per cent said that they would like to extend their role in the surgery. On the other hand, 51 per cent said they felt that the performance of delegated medical tasks was not within the role of the nurse.

Perhaps the uncertainty expressed in the conflicting views forwarded by some nurses reflects the current uncertain position of nursing as a profession. Nursing bodies are still attempting to produce a unique definition of the role of the nurse and an independent body of knowledge to support it. The data presented indicated that nurses were uncertain of their role. District nurses in particular appeared to cling to the traditional definitions of their role. It would be expected that these nurses would show more role uncertainty than treatment room nurses when faced with the issue of delegation. In their own defence they argue that their role is caring for the patient, which often meant bathing and dressing. But, as other nurses pointed out, nursing is changing. Different types of nurse specialist are emerging. District nurses are transferring more work to the surgery and may even assist the doctor. Although Reedy and his colleagues (1980b) found that such nurses generally felt that this trend was a good thing, the role of the district nurse is inevitably questioned. This threat may be enhanced by the increasing number of untrained staff, such as nursing auxiliaries or bath attendants, performing tasks which district nurses once performed – and often still do. As long as the debate over the role of the nurse continues, the debate over delegation will continue.

One main problem of nurses undertaking an expanded role in the surgery is their lack of preparatory training. Treatment room nurses were as likely as district nurses to feel inadequately trained for such a role. Many treatment room nurses said they entered this branch of nursing because of the flexible working hours which suited their family commitments, rather than for any professional reasons. Although the necessity to work flexible hours among women with small children may ensure an adequate supply of applicants for treatment room posts, professional recognition and the systematic organization of such work may attract more nurses. It may also attract more nurses with a commitment to developing nursing as a profession, and hence with a commitment to the nurse practitioner role rather than that of a doctor's assistant. However, such a role can be developed in a way professionally acceptable to nursing only if all treatment room nurses are responsible to other, more senior, nurses, rather than to the doctors by whom they are usually employed. This can become possible only if these nurses are uniformly employed by the health authorities and attached to practices in the same way as district nurses and treatment room nurses working in health centres. Doctors would undoubtedly be opposed to this scheme as they would lose control over the nurse. Lack of control over ancillary staff was one of the main reasons doctors in this survey gave for opposing health centre practice.

In conclusion, in its efforts to achieve professional status, nursing is attempting to achieve an identity independent of medicine. The current debate on the role of the nurse was reflected in respondents' attitudes towards undertaking delegated medical tasks. If nurses undertake more medical functions, then they are identifying themselves even more closely with medicine. This makes it difficult for nursing to satisfy all the prerequisites of professional status. However, the concern with professional status and the role of the nurse places more, not less, urgency on the development of a nurse practitioner role in general practice, otherwise nurses working with general practitioners may well be consumed by medicine and simply become doctors' assistants.

10

DISCUSSION

So what is the future for delegation and for doctors and nurses
working in primary care? The Report of the Royal Commission on
Medical Education (1968) stated that general practitioners should be
freed from routine trivial work not requiring their level of skill and
expertise. It appears from this study, and from the ratio of doctors to
treatment room nurses nationally, that this has not yet occurred. This
research indicates that while most doctors and nurses are in favour of
expanding the clinical role of the nurse in the surgery, reservations
continue to exist concerning the delegation of diagnostic procedures.
Moreover, a significant minority both of doctors and nurses even
expressed misgivings about an expanded clinical role for nurses.
However, treatment room nurses were more positively orientated
towards the performance of more clinical procedures, and younger
nurses were more enthusiastic about undertaking diagnostic functions. This allows a certain degree of optimism for future developments
in this field.

This research also indicates that as more recent graduates replace
older doctors, as more doctors practise from groups and take an
interest in more efficient methods of practice organization and in
undertaking a wider range of activities, then delegation may be
practised more extensively. Although no evidence was found to
suggest that attitudes towards delegating initial screening in the
surgery will change as more young doctors enter general practice, the
findings do suggest that the more doctors delegate then the more
favourable their attitudes will be towards this practice. Thus, age may
be related indirectly. Other research has also indicated that attitudes
may change with an improvement in communication between health
care professionals (Miller and Backett 1980).

The challenge for the future, then, is how to develop the clinical and diagnostic aspect of the treatment room nurse's role, while minimizing role conflict and overlap between doctors and nurses. Doctors' opposition towards delegating part of their role is not unexpected in view of their history of role and status insecurity. Earlier chapters showed that each step doctors took towards becoming members of the medical profession was at the expense of accepting a reduction in status. Similarly, nurses' opposition towards undertaking medical procedures is not unexpected in view of their current attempts to develop an independent body of knowledge. As role changes within one occupation inevitably have repercussions on the structure of closely related occupations, attempts to delegate the procedures belonging to one group to another are inevitably going to be viewed with some degree of suspicion. The nursing profession is forced by this debate to decide whether it is in its interests to undertake delegated medical tasks and whether an expanded nurse role can be developed in a way which does not conflict with nursing's professional aspirations. If nurses are to expand their role, this implies that they must be explicit about their current roles in order to initiate and develop changes within the model of nursing. Similarly, if general practitioners are to delegate part of their current role then they must work with a clear definition of general practice.

Such role changes must be effected with a great deal of thought and planning in order not to conflict with professional interests. But how are occupational changes normally effected? In the past the delegation of routine tasks has occurred during phases of medical advance and thus during periods when it is likely to be perceived as less threatening to the medical profession. Similarly, in the past nurses were not so concerned about not performing the tasks belonging to another profession. For example, the taking of temperatures, once a medical procedure, became less important to doctors in an era of changing medical knowledge and gradually became delegated to nurses. Tasks are not simply delegated because they become routine or too numerous. Advantages have to be seen in their delegation, particularly by the delegator. Both the medical and nursing professions need convincing that the role changes which accompany a more extensive degree of delegation are not necessarily bad. More research demonstrating this is necessary. For example, it has been demonstrated (Scherer *et al.* 1977) that doctors working with nurse practitioners report that their roles change in a positive way. At the same time as increasing their list sizes, they spend more time with patients with complicated medical problems and give less routine patient care. Nurses undertaking a nurse practitioner role also find that it is not the nature of their role which changes, rather that there is an increase in the complexity of the tasks they perform and in their level of clinical judgement (Yeomans 1977).

Of course, for any occupation to change a favourable social climate is also needed. For example, the Medical Act of 1848 was partly the result of the spirit of reform and the desire to eliminate corruption and élitism. The development of nursing as a respectable occupation received impetus from the emancipation of women. In the future, it is possible that role changes in both medicine and nursing may be effected by the current emphasis on preventive medicine and the changing morbidity and mortality structure of the population. Changes in inter-professional relationships may be increasingly seen as necessary for the promotion of health.

Despite the suggestion that increasing the prestige value of innovations encourages their development, the issue is more complex than this (Becker 1970). Although general practitioners have always been reluctant to delegate due to their narrow conceptions of independence, their isolation from medical technology, even in an era when such technology is being questioned, may make them more reluctant to delegate part of their role.

The doctors interviewed often expressed a fear that more delegation would result in a loss of independence and detract from their role. If doctors are to be encouraged to delegate extensively then they must see that the advantages outweigh the disadvantages. They must not feel threatened. This implies the development of a clearly defined role, no longer based on superficial descriptions and no longer depending on a narrow definition of independence. Several areas in which doctors might concentrate have been suggested: preventive medicine including involvement in community action as well as attention to individuals, emotional aspects of illness, and developing the clinical aspects of their work.

Little indication emerged from the present study on the direction general practice might take in the future. Most doctors interviewed simply saw their role in terms of being the person of first contact in health care and as 'sorting out the major from the minor'. Although 59 per cent maintained that their role included the treatment of emotional problems, many general practitioners added that this was only because there was no one else available to dispense such treatment. Nor were recent graduates any more likely to be interested in this branch of medicine. With regard to the clinical aspects of their role, few doctors felt enthusiastic about this although they were willing to undertake more minor surgical procedures given the financial incentive to do so, better facilities and more time. Unfortunately, preventive medicine was not covered by the interview schedule used and the issue was rarely raised by the doctors interviewed. Each of the areas of role development suggested are arguably in the public interest, although greater concentration on prevention is likely to result in a better equilibrium between input and output in medical care. There is no reason why general practitioners could not simultaneously develop each aspect: involvement with emotional aspects of illness, clinical procedures, and preventive medicine. It is doubtful whether concentration on clinical aspects of medicine alone would give general practitioners their desired unique body of knowledge, as this really is an extension of hospital medicine. Possibly the most profitable area to be examined, especially from the point of view of the public, is a more radical approach to prevention. For example, how can doctors help communities to help themselves in the area of health? How can doctors fight commercial and political pressures inducing ill health? How can doctors help to change social environments? Those doctors concerned with answering such questions may find some insight in Rosenthal's (1980) descriptions of community approaches to health in which lay health workers have been employed, for example by community health councils, to raise health issues locally. Their aims included the stimulation of greater awareness of the meaning of health and of the causes of ill health. The involvement of the general practitioner in such schemes was fairly significant. Meetings with general practitioners and hospital doctors were held and they became included in discussions with the public on a broad range of health issues. So far, community health projects have had little contact with environmental health issues, limiting themselves to lead pollution and health and safety at work. However, they are still in their early days.

Of course, such community-based projects inevitably threaten the traditional monopoly of health held by the medical profession. The question is how to deal with any consequent hostility and how to minimize doctor opposition. The solution, as with delegation, must lie partly in medical education. Medical education does not even adequately equip general practitioners to deal with their currently ill-defined role. For example, a survey of medical graduates from Aberdeen University, ten to twelve years after graduation, showed that a substantial majority favoured the development of formal undergraduate training in general practice and a third said that much of their medical education was obsolete (McAndrew, Dawson and

Ogston 1970). Planning effective medical education for general practitioners requires a clear, well-defined concept of the functions and organizational structure of primary care and of the roles of the professionals within it. No magical answers can be given, as is evident from the collection of papers on medical education and primary care edited by Noack (1980). However, questions which appear worth concentrating on include: how can medical students learn to establish fruitful relationships with their patients, encourage them to ask questions, and educate them in health and health promotion; how to be interested in dealing with emotional anxieties; and how to resist feelings of omnipotence and to fight the pressures creating ill health. It is relevant to ask what contribution can the sociologist make towards these aims?

Changes in the age structure of the population, in the nature of diseases, and the priorities attached to various aspects of health care by the Department of Health may, in any case, have an effect on professional roles. For example, the contrast between the increasing expenditure on technological medicine and its diminishing returns has already been pointed out. Although mortality rates have drama-tically declined since the 1800s, this has been largely due to improved sanitation and nutritional standards. The current diseases of indust-rialized societies are largely products of these societies. If the environment is polluted, housing and conditions of work poor, and if inappropriate life styles and nutritional habits are encouraged, for example by advertising, then output will not necessarily equal input into the National Health Service. Indeed, a recent report by the Department of Health and Social Security (1980a) quite clearly states that social class differences in health are as great today as in 1948. In essence, it indicates that the British working class are much more likely to suffer from ill health and die before retirement than the professional class, and the gap is as large as when the National Health Service was first inaugurated. Not only does this Report indicate that poverty must be eliminated and social conditions changed, but that the quality and quantity of health care facilities needs increasing. However, to improve services requires financial outlays, and at a time of increasing cuts in government expenditure such resources are unlikely to be forthcoming. Even if the financial savings from the elimination of the area health authorities were to be redirected into service provision this is unlikely to be sufficient. Here again, a partial solution to the problem is an increased amount of delegation, and the development of an extended nurse role – a role which would include not only treatment, but a commitment to health education and preventive medicine, alongside general practitioners.

Nurses could play a far larger role in primary care if caring and prevention or patient education were emphasized instead of merely the treatment of ill health. If nurses could be seen to be making a valuable contribution to health care in their own right, the nursing profession might be less reluctant to permit them to simultaneously undertake medical functions. The Department of Health's priorities for the National Health Service emphasize the importance of services for the elderly, the mentally ill, and mentally handicapped, as well as for children. On the whole, emphasis is placed on those with chronic conditions who make high demands on the health service (Department of Health and Social Security 1976c; 1977a). Nurses could easily extend their role to encompass the provision of treatment for such groups and the education of these patients in health matters may be a worthwhile area of endeavour.

Inevitably, doctors and nurses would need to work together closely, and there may be a certain degree of role overlap. However, while different groups of professionals are working together for the benefit of the patient there can be no escape from a certain degree of overlap. Such suggestions are by no means innovatory. The increasing shift towards health rather than sickness care implies a movement towards patient education, screening, prevention and more involvement in the management of chronic illness. The emphasis on the elderly, for example, has simulated some general practitioners to set up age/sex registers. Health visitors and district nurses have been active in assessing the health of elderly patients on those registers (Williamson 1970; Wallace 1975). Only a slight change of emphasis is needed to progress from this to the role of the nurse practitioner who makes diagnostic assessments, carries out treatments, and imparts health education. Such an intermediate role, of course, would also have the benefit of reducing the gap between the medically qualified and the layman.

For nurses to be encouraged to expand their role in primary care the benefits to nursing must be emphasized. The fact that nurses would simply be expanding a role which already exists rather than introducing anything new has to be stressed. Nurses also need convincing that their unique caring role will be a central part of an expanded role. Certainly, nurse practitioners, because of the caring element of their role, are perceived as remaining nurses while extending and adding a medical component to their work. While nurse practitioners working alongside traditional nurses in the United States report quite different patterns of work, this is not because they do different things but rather due to the fact that they give more systematic assessments and a higher priority to health education (Yeomans 1977). Furthermore, unlike many treatment room nurses in Britain, nurse practitioners in the United States are not employed by doctors, but by institutions – they are also responsible to other nurses. Moreover, in many states of America nurse practitioners are legally entitled to act independently without any medical supervision. Research has shown that nurse practitioners certainly do not see themselves simply as substitute doctors (Linn 1974). Nursing organizations in this country need to be convinced that similar steps could be taken here to help ensure that an expanded role for nurses in general practice would not hinder the question for autonomy among nurses.

It is unfortunate that debate often revolves around professional disputes rather than the proposition that overqualification is wasteful and unproductive. There appears to be a need for a more consumer-centred health service concerned with the needs of practice, rather than the needs of professional status. At present it is insufficient to point out to many doctors and nurses that the practice of delegation may result in a more efficient system of health care and to positive changes in roles. Many doctors are reluctant to practise delegation on an extensive scale, including diagnostic as well as clinical tasks, and not all nurses are willing or able to undertake these tasks. However, as doctors and treatment room nurses held more favourable views towards an extended clinical, if not diagnostic, role, it appears that there is a need for the setting up of uniform training courses which would be mandatory for nurses wanting to work in doctors' surgeries. This need is particularly pressing as most nurses felt untrained for an extended role and many treatment room nurses' education in the performance of tasks such as ear syringing was limited to instruction from the doctors they worked with. However, there is little likelihood of such mandatory courses being set up in the near future. Not only has the idea been recently rejected by the Joint Board for Clinical Nursing Studies, but educational changes are also invariably slow. For example, training for district nurses, a long-established branch of nursing, only becomes mandatory from 1981. Similarly, vocational training for general practitioners themselves does not become mandatory until 1981. However, if nurses continue to perform delegated medical tasks in an unsystematic and unrecognized way, with no education in their theoretical bases, then confusion over legal responsibilities and legitimate roles will continue. Until the role of the treatment room nurse is properly recognized it is difficult to see how a nurse practitioner role can even begin to be introduced into British primary care.

Of course, there is currently an additional handicap to increased delegation: fears of doctor unemployment. This means that schemes including the substitution of medical for non-medical labour will meet with greater opposition from doctors. On the other hand, the present controversy over a surplus of doctors is partly artificial as it is to a certain degree due to the cutbacks in public expenditure resulting in the freezing of posts. Furthermore, the continuous cycle of shortages to surpluses of doctors calls for better, and more realistic, manpower planning, taking account of the possibilities for the substitution of labour. It is unlikely that either nurse practitioners or physicians' assistants will be introduced into British primary care in the near future. However, in view of our precarious history of manpower planning, this does not mean that they may not be needed simply because of a future shortage of doctors. The fact also remains that, even in times of an over-supply of doctors, it is inefficient to encourage personnel to perform tasks for which they are overqualified.

Initial resistance to a more extensive degree of delegation involving the inclusion of diagnostic techniques does not imply that experiments involving nurse practitioners in British primary care cannot be embarked upon. One experimental scheme has already been completed (Reedy, Stewart, and Quick 1980). These authors have studied an experiment in an English health centre including four general practitioners, their ancillary staff, and a final-year physician's associate from Duke University in North Carolina. The associate was attached to the practice for a period of approximately eight weeks and managed 221 cases, mainly common acute problems, under the supervision of the doctors. The doctors in the practice were unanimous in saying that the experiment had worked very well and had been entirely acceptable to patients. However, they were doubtful if the organizational upheaval caused by creating a new group of health care personnel was warranted on a large scale. On the other hand, the authors certainly felt that it would be possible to train such auxiliary personnel in the United Kingdom, who could be trusted to cope with a large proportion of straightforward medical problems and refer more difficult cases to the doctor.

Logically, the next development should be the initiation of similar experiments in a number of general practices with nurses who have been given further training to equip them for such a role. This would include evaluation studies of task performance, the quality and quantity of care given together with outcome measures, cost–benefit analyses, and measures of patient and professional satisfaction. If such experiments prove to be successful then it should be easier to encourage the more widespread adoption of such a scheme. Fears and prejudices may be overcome as both health professionals and the public become more familiar with the system. However, before such a system could be adopted in a widespread way not only does professional resistance have to be overcome but larger group practice, better premises, and even greater practice from health centres, together with a greater degree of teamwork, needs to be encouraged. Such changes are occurring slowly, but a new generation of doctors may be needed before they occur more rapidly.

What about the policy of the Department of Health and Social Security? Is it likely to encourage such a restructuring of general practice? Although the recent Royal Commission on the National Health Service commissioned a study of the literature on nurse practitioners by MacGuire (1980), their report of 1979 concluded that they saw no place for such personnel in this country. This conclusion is inexplicable in view of MacGuire's positive conclusions concerning nurse practitioners. The report feebly encouraged an expanded clinical role for existing nurses as long as their caring role did not suffer. However, as no definitions of an expanded nurse role were offered the report, in effect, offered little guidance.

How does the present economic climate affect the possible adoption of a policy encouraging delegation? Public funds allocated to the health service are inevitably affected by the economic circumstances of the nation. Although health expenditure has been increasing in real terms almost continuously since 1949, the mid-1970s onwards has seen constraints on public spending. The National Health Service itself does not appear to be in danger of being dismantled, only certain segments of its structure such as the area health authorities. However, the National Health Service not only has a very large labour force, but also one that is becoming increasingly expensive. This alone indicates a need for labour-saving devices which increase productivity and is one point in favour of the substitution of medical labour for less costly personnel. As has been previously noted, few adequate cost–benefit analyses have been done in this field. However, McTernan (1976) has estimated that the cost of training a physician's assistant or nurse practitioner is half that of training a doctor and also takes half the time. In addition, the costs of turning a nurse into a nurse practitioner are relatively small. On the other hand, as with the introduction of any new system, substantial financial outlays are needed at the outset, particularly in the establishing of special training courses. A period of economic growth will probably be needed before the British Government would be willing to adopt such a scheme. Nevertheless, there is no reason why a smaller financial outlay could not be made for the purposes of experimentation. It cannot be over-emphasized that roles need to be adapted to changing conditions (Ferguson 1973). Initial experimental schemes may encourage and facilitate such developments.

To sum up, the success of a scheme involving the introduction of nurse practitioners cannot be guaranteed without the co-operation and support of both the medical and nursing professions. At present this is forthcoming only in an extremely limited sense, because of concerns with professional status. Perhaps the question which really needs analysis is: why professionalize if it only creates divisions and conflicts and is not always in the public interest? Part of the answer lies in McKnight's definition of professionalism:

> 'We need to solve your problems
> We need to tell you what they are
> We need to deal with them in our terms
> We need to have you respect our satisfaction with our own work.'
>
> (McKnight 1977: 89)

REFERENCES

Abel, R. A. (1969) *Nursing Attachments to General Practice*. London: HMSO.

Abel Smith, B. (1960) *A History of the Nursing Profession*. London: Heinemann.

Abel Smith, B. and Gales, K. (1964) *British Doctors at Home and Abroad*. London: Bell and Sons. Occasional Papers in Social Administration No. 8.

American Medical Association News (1970) AMA Urges Major New Role for Nurses. November 25: 1–8.

American Nurses Association (1971) *The American Nurses Association Views the Emerging Physician's Assistant*. New York: The Association.

Anderson, O. W. (1968) *Towards an Unambiguous Profession? A Review of Nursing*. University of Chicago: Health Administration Perspectives No. A6.

Annandale Steiner, D. (1979) Unhappiness is the Nurse who Expected More. *Nursing Mirror* November 29: 34–6.

Bailit, H., Lewis, J., Hochheiser, L., and Bush, N. (1975) Assessing the Quality of Care. *Nursing Outlook* **23**: 153–59.

Balint, M. (1957) *The Doctor, his Patient and the Illness*. London: Pitman Medical.

Balint, M. and Balint, E. (1961) *Psychotherapeutic Techniques in Medicine*. London: Tavistock. Mind and Medicine Monographs No. 1.

Barber, J. H. (1971) Computer Assisted Recording in General Practice. *Journal of the Royal College of General Practitioners* **21**: 726–36.

Beck, R. G. (1971) Viewpoint of the Consumer. In *Report of the Proceedings of National Conference on Assistant to the Physician*. Department of Health and Welfare, Canada.

Becker, M. H. (1970). Factors Affecting Diffusion of Innovations among Health Professionals. *American Journal of Public Health* **60** 294–304.

Berkowitz, N. and Malone, M. F. (1968) Intraprofessional Conflict. *Nursing Forum* **1**: 50–71.

Berlant, J. (1975) *Profession and Monopoly*. Berkely: University of California Press.

Bessman, A. N. (1974) Comparison of Medical Care in Nurse Clinician and Physician Clinics in Medical School Affiliated Hospitals. *Journal of Chronic Diseases* **27**: 115–25.

Boddy, F. A. (1969) General Practitioners View the Home Nursing Service. *British Medical Journal* **ii**: 438–41.

Bonnet, P. D. (1972) Medical Care in the United States. In J. Fry and W. Farndale (eds) *International Medical Care*. Oxford: Medical and Technical Publishing.

Borland, B. (1972) A Survey of Attitudes of Physicians on Proper Use of Physician Assistants. *Health Services Review* **87**: 467–72.

Bowling, A. (1980a) Who's Afraid of the Paramedic? *World Medicine* June 28: 48.

— (1980b) To do or not to do? *Nursing Mirror* July 17: 30–2.

— (1980c) Diagnosis is the Doctor's Job. *Mims Magazine* September 1: 51–6.

— (1980d) Nurses in the Primary Care Team. *Lancet* **ii**: 590.

— (1980e) A Nurse Practitioner in Britain? *Nursing Times* December 4: 2157–158.

Breytspraak, L. M. and Pondy, L. R. (1969) Sociological Evaluation of the Physician's Assistant Role Relations. *Group Practice* March: 32–41.

British Medical Association (1950) *General Practice and the Training of the General Practitioner*. Report of a Committee of the Association.

— (1974) *Primary Health Care Teams*. Board of Science and Education.

— (1977) Evidence to the Royal Commission on the National Health Service. *British Medical Journal* **i**: 314–16.

Buchan, I. C. and Richardson, I. M. (1973) *Time Study of Consultations in General Practice*. Edinburgh: Scottish Home and Health Department. Scottish Home Service Studies No. 27.

Butler, J. R. (1980) *How Many Patients?* London: Bedford Square Press. Occasional Papers on Social Administration No. 64.

Butler, J. R., Bevan, J. M., and Taylor, R. C. (1973) *Family Doctors and Public Policy*. London: Routledge and Kegan Paul.

Butterfield, J. and Wadsworth, M. (1966) A London Teaching Hospital. In G. McLachlan (ed.) *Problems and Progress in Medical*

Care. Published for the Nuffield Provincial Hospitals Trust by Oxford University Press.

Canadian Nurses Association (1970) *Statement on the Expanded Role of the Nurse. Part Two: The Physician's Assistant.* (Unpublished.)

Cartwright, A. (1967) *Patients and their Doctors.* London: Routledge and Kegan Paul.

Cartwright, A. and O'Brien, M. (1976) Social Class Variations in Health Care and in the Nature of General Practitioner Consultations. In M. Stacey (ed.) *The Sociology of the NHS.* Sociological Review Monograph **22**: 77–98.

Cartwright, A. and Anderson, R. (1981) *General Practice Revisited.* London: Tavistock.

Clyne, M. R. (1974) How Personal is Care in General Practice? *Journal of the Royal College of General Practitioners* **24**: 263.

Collings, J. S. (1950) General Practice in England Today, A Reconnaissance. *Lancet* **i**: 555.

Conant, L. (1974) The Nurse's View. In D. M. Pitcairn and D. Flahault (eds) *The Medical Assistant.* World Health Organisation, Public Health Papers no. 60.

Cornelius, D. (1970) ANA Reaction. *American Medical Association News* November 25: 7.

Coy, R. D. and Hansen, M. F. (1969) The Doctor's Assistant: A Survey of Physicians' Expectations. *Journal of the American Medical Association* **209**: 529–33.

Cunningham, D. J., Bevan, J. M., and Floyd, C. B. (1972) The Role of the Practice Nurse from the Patient's Point of View. *Community Medicine* **128**: 534–38.

Curwen, M. H. (1964) Lord Moran's Ladder. *Journal of the Royal College of General Practitioners* **7**: 38–65.

Dajda, R. (1980) Who Presents? The Illusion of Power Sharing in the Surgery. In R. Mapes (ed.) *Prescribing Practice and Drug Usage.* London: Croom Helm.

Dan Mason Nursing Research Committee of the National Florence Nightingale Memorial Committee (1967) *Marriage and Nursing – A Survey of Registered and Enrolled Nurses.*

Davies, C. (1978) Four Events in Nursing History: A New Look. *Nursing Times Occasional Papers* 74, No. 17.

Department of Health and Social Security. *Annual Reports.* 1950–1977.
— (1971) *International Certificates of Vaccination against Smallpox and Cholera.* Health Circular 14/70.

— (1974) *Health and Personal Social Service Statistics for England.* London: HMSO.

— (1975) *Nurses Employed Privately by General Medical Practitioners.* Staff Training Memorandum (75) 13.

— (1976a) *Prevention and Health: Everybody's Business.* London: HMSO.

— (1976b) *Vaccination and Immunisation – Involvement of Nursing Staff.* Health Circular (76) 26.

— (1976c) *Priorities for Health and Personal Social Services.* London: HMSO.

— (1977a) *The Way Forward: Priorities in the Health and Social Services.* London: HMSO.

— (1977b) *The Extending Role of the Clinical Nurse.* Legal Implications and Training Requirements. Health Circular (77) 22.

— (1978) *Medical Manpower in the Next Twenty Years.* London: HMSO.

— (1980a) *Inequalities in Health.* London: HMSO.

— (1980b) *Health and Personal Social Services Statistics for England 1978.* London: HMSO.

Department of Health and Welfare, Canada (1971) *Report of the Proceedings of National Conference on Assistant to the Physician.*

Dingwall, R. (1976) Accomplishing Profession. *Sociological Review* **24**: 331–50.

Dolan, M. B. (1969) *More Nurses, Better Nursing.* Paper Presented at Nursing Biennial Convention, Detroit. (Unpublished.)

Drury, M. (1977) Premises and Organisation. In J. Fry (ed.) *Trends in General Practice 1977.* Published for the Royal College of General Practitioners by the British Medical Association.

Drury, M. and Kuenssberg, E. V. (1970) Inquiry into Administrative Activities in General Practice. *British Medical Journal* **iv**: 42–4.

Dunnell, K. and Cartwright, C. (1972) *Medicine Takers, Prescribers and Hoarders.* London: Routledge and Kegan Paul.

Eichenberger, R., Hume, W., Watson, K., and Hawkins, R. (1970) Kentucky Physicians' Response to a New Health Professional. *Journal of the Kentucky Medical Association* May: 303–10.

Eimerl, T. S. and Pearson, R. J. C. (1968) Working Time in General Practice: How General Practitioners Use Their Time. *British Medical Journal* **ii**: 1549–554.

Elliot Dixon, J. (1970) *Ask the Man who Uses One.* Third Annual Duke Conference on Physician's Assistants. Duke University, North Carolina.

Estes, E. H. (1969) Task Oriented versus Degree Oriented Training. *Military Medicine* **134**: 386.

Etzioni, A. (1969) *The Semi-Professions and their Organizations: Teachers, Nurses and Social Workers.* New York: The Free Press.

Facts about Nursing, 1972–1973. American Nurses Association.

Fairweather, J. C. and Kifolo, A. (1972) Improvement of Patient Care in a Solo OB-GYN Practice by using an RN Physician's Assistant. *American Journal of Public Health* **62**: 361–63.

Fendall, N. R. E. (1972) Auxiliaries and Primary Medical Care. *Bulletin of the New York Academy of Medicine* **48**: 1291–300.

Ferguson, M. (1973) Nurse or Feldsher? A Crisis of Identity. *Nursing Times* October 25: 1410–412.

Forsyth, G. and Logan, R. F. L. (1968) *Gateway or Dividing Line?* Published for the Nuffield Provincial Hospitals Trust by Oxford University Press.

Fottler, M., Gibson, G., and Pinchoff, D. (1978) Physicians' Attitudes Towards the Nurse Practitioner. *Journal of Health and Social Behaviour* **19**: 303–11.

Freidson, E. (1970) *Profession of Medicine.* New York: Dodd Mead and Co.

— Para-medical Personnel. *International Encyclopedia of Social Science*, Vol. 10: 114–20.

Fritz, E. and Murphy, M. (1966) An Analysis of the Positions of Nursing Education. *Nursing Outlook* February 14: 20–4.

Fry, L. (1960) Casualties and Casuals. *Lancet* i: 163.

Fry, J. (1972) Twenty One Years of General Practice – Changing Patterns. *Journal of the Royal College of General Practitioners* **22**: 521–28.

— (1974) *Common Diseases: Their Nature, Incidence and Care.* London: Medical and Technical Publishing.

— (1977) The Place of Primary Care. In J. Fry (ed.) *Trends in General Practice 1977.* Published for the Royal College of General Practitioners by the British Medical Association.

Gemmill, P. F. (1958) An American Report on the NHS. *British Medical Journal*, Supplement July 5: 17.

Gilmore, M., Bruce, N., and Hunt, M. (1974) *The Work of the Nursing Team in General Practice.* Council for the Education and Training of Health Visitors.

Goldberg, E. M. and Neill, J. (1972) *Social Work in General Practice.* London: George Allen and Unwin.

Goldie, N. (1977) The Division of Labour among the Mental Health

Professions – A Negotiated or an Imposed Order. In M. Stacey, M. Reid, C. Heath, and R. Dingwall (eds) *Health and the Division of Labour.* London: Croom Helm.

Gray, Pereira D. J. (1980) Just a GP. *Journal of the Royal College of General Practitioners* **30**: 231–39.

Gunawardena, A. and Lee, K. (1977) Access and Efficiency in Medical Care. In K. Barnard and K. Lee (eds) *Conflicts in the NHS.* London: Croom Helm.

Hadfield, S. J. (1953) A Field Survey of General Practice 1951–1952. *British Medical Journal* **i**: 683–706.

Hadley, R. T. I. (1976) Idaho Nurse brings Enthusiasm to State Post. *American Nurse* **8**: 31.

Hasler, J. C., Hemphill, P. M. R., Stewart, T. I., Boyle, N., Harris, A., and Palmer, E. (1968) Development of the Nursing Section of the Community Health Team. *British Medical Journal* **iii**: 734–36.

Hasler, J. C., Greenland, A. S., Jacka, S. M., Prichard, P. M. M., and Reedy, B. L. E. C. (1972) Training for the Treatment Room Sister in General Practice. *British Medical Journal* **i**: 232–34.

Hasler, J. C. and Klinger, M. (1976) Common Ground in General Practitioner and Health Visitor Training – An Experimental Course. *Journal of the Royal College of General Practitioners* **26**: 266–76.

Hector, W. (1973) *Mrs Bedford Fenwick.* London: Royal College of Nursing.

Heiman, E. M. and Dempsey, M. K. (1976) Independent Behaviour of Nurse Practitioners: A Survey of Physician and Nurse Attitudes. *American Journal of Public Health* **66**: 587–89.

Henderson, V. (1967) *The Nature of Nursing.* London: Collier-Macmillan.

Hicks, D. (1976) *Primary Health Care.* London: HMSO.

Hockey, L. (1968) *Care in the Balance.* London: Queen's Institute of District Nursing.

Hodgkin, G. K. H. (1967) Saving a Doctor's Time with a Practice Nurse. In E. V. Kuenssberg (ed.) *Conference Report: The Team. Family Health Care.* Royal College of General Practitioners.

Hodgkin, G. K. H. and Gillie, C. (1968) Relieving the Strain by Work Study and a Practice Nurse in a Two Doctor Urban Practice. In The Practice Nurse. *Journal of the Royal College of General Practitioners. Reports from General Practice* X.

Holloway, S. W. F. (1966) The Apothecaries Act 1815: A Reinterpretation. *Medical History* Part I: 107–29; Part II: 221–36.

Holohan, A. M., Newell, D. J., and Walker, J. H. (1975) Practitioners, Patients and the Accident Department. *Hospital and Health Services Review* **71**, 3: 80–3.

Holohan, A. M. (1976) Accident and Emergency Departments. Illness and Accident Behaviour. In M. Stacey (ed.) *The Sociology of the NHS*. Sociological Review Monograph No. 22.

Honigsbaum, F. (1972) Quality in General Practice. *Journal of the Royal College of General Practitioners* **22**: 429.

Horder, J. P. (1977) Physicians and Family Doctors: A New Relationship. *Journal of the Royal College of General Practitioners* **27**: 391–97.

Hospital Plan. National Health Service (1962). London: HMSO.

Hospital Plan. National Health Service (1966). London: HMSO.

House, V. (1977) Attitudes to Degree Courses and Shortened Courses for Graduates. *Nursing Times Occasional Paper* March 31.

Howie, J. (1977) Patterns of Work. In J. Fry (ed) *Trends in General Practice 1977*. Published for the Royal College of General Practitioners by the British Medical Association.

Hughes, E. C., Hughes, E., and Deutscher, I. (1958) *Twenty Thousand Nurses Tell their Story*. Philadelphia: Lippincott and Co.

Hull, F. M. (1972) Diagnostic Pathways in General Practice. *Journal of the Royal College of General Practitioners* **22**: 241–58.

Hunt, M. (1972) The Dilemma of Identity in Health Visiting. *Nursing Times* **68**, Supplement: 17–20; 23–4.

Illich, I. (1975) *Medical Nemesis*. London: Calder and Boyars.

— (1977) Disabling Professions. In I. Illich, I. Zola, J. McKnight, J. Caplan, and H. Shaiken (eds) *Disabling Professions*. London: Marion Boyars.

Interim Report on the Future Provision of Medical and Allied Services (1920) (Dawson Committee). London: HMSO.

Irvine, D. and Jefferys, M. (1971) British Medical Association Planning Unit Survey of General Practice 1969. *British Medical Journal* **iv**: 535–43.

Israel, S. and Draper, P. (1971) General Practitioner Hospital Beds: A Review. *British Medical Journal* **i**: 452–56.

Jefferys, M. (1965) *Anatomy of Social Welfare Services*. London: Michael Joseph.

Johnson, T. (1972) *Professions and Power*. London: Macmillan.

Joint Board of Clinical Nursing Studies (1978) The Extending Role of the Clinical Nurse. *Bulletin* No. 18, Summer.

Joint Committee on Postgraduate Training for General Practice

180   *Delegation in General Practice*

(1976) *Criteria for the Selection of General Practitioner Trainers*. London: JCPTGP.
Journal of the Royal College of General Practitioners (1972) How Many Patients? **22**: 491–93.

Komaroff, A. L., Black, W. L., Flatley, M., Knopp, R. H., Reiffen, B., and Sherman, H. (1974) Protocols for Physician's Assistants. *New England Journal of Medicine* **290**: 307–12.
Kuenssberg, E. V. (1971) General Practice Through the Looking Glass. *The Practitioner* **206**: 129–45.
Kurtz, R. A. and Flaming, K. H. (1963) Professionalism: The Case of Nurses. *American Journal of Nursing* **63**: 75–9.

Lancet (1974) Editorial. A Nurse Practitioner **i**: 608–09.
Last, J. M., Martin, F. M., and Stanley, G. R. (1967) Academic Record and Subsequent Career. *Proceedings of the Royal Society of Medicine* **60**: 813–16.
Last, J. M. and Stanley, G. R. (1968) Career Preferences of Young British Doctors. *British Journal of Medical Education* **2**: 137–55.
Lawrence, R. S., DeFriese, G. H., Putnam, S. M., Pickard, C. G., Cyr, A. B., and Whiteside, S. W. (1977) Physician Receptivity to Nurse Practitioners. *Medical Care* **XV**: 298–310.
Linn, L. S. (1974) Care vs. Cure. How the Nurse Practitioner Views the Patient. *Nursing Outlook* **22**: 641–44.
— (1976) Patient Acceptance of the Family Nurse Practitioner. *Medical Care* **14**: 357–64.
Litman, T. J. (1972) Public Perceptions of the Physician's Assistant. *American Journal of Public Health* **62**: 343–46.
Long, A. and Atkins, J. B. (1974) Communications between General Practitioners and Consultants. *British Medical Journal* **iv**: 456–59.
Loudon, I. (1977) The General Practitioner and the Hospital. In J. Fry (ed.) *Trends in General Practice 1977*. Published for the Royal College of General Practitioners by the British Medical Association.
Lysaught, J. P. L. (1974) *Action in Nursing*. New York: McGraw Hill.

MacGuire, J. (1969) *Threshold to Nursing*. London: Bell and Sons. Occasional Paper in Social Administration No. 30.
— (1980) *The Expanded Role of the Nurse*. London: King Edward's Hospital Fund for London.
Malone, M. (1961) The Paradox in Nursing. *American Journal of Nursing* **9**: 52–5.

— (1964) The Dilemma of a Professional in a Bureaucracy. *Nursing Forum* **4**: 36–60.

Marsh, G. N. (1969) Visiting Nurse – Analysis of One Year's Work. *British Medical Journal* **iv**: 42–4.

Marsh, G. N. and McRay, R. A. (1974) Team Work in an English Practice. *British Medical Journal* **i**: 319.

Marsh, G. N. and Kaim Caudle, P. (1976) *Team Care in General Practice*. London: Croom Helm.

Matteson, T. and Smith; S. V. (1977) Medical Speciality Choice. A Note on Status Rankings. *Social Science and Medicine* **11**: 421–23.

Maynard, A. and Walker, A. (1977) Too Many Doctors? *Lloyds Bank Review* **125**: 24–36.

— (1978) *Doctor Manpower 1975–2000: Alternative Forecasts and their Resource Implications*. A Report for the Royal Commission on the National Health Service. London: HMSO.

McAndrew, G. M., Dawson, A. A., and Ogston, D. (1970) The Undergraduate Curriculum in Retrospect. *British Journal of Medical Education* **48**: 323–31.

McCormack, R. C. and Crawford, R. L. (1971) Attitudes of Professional Nurses Toward Primary Care. In E. P Lewis (ed.) *Changing Patterns of Nursing Practice: New Needs, New Roles*. New York: American Journal of Nursing Co.

McIntosh, J. and Dingwall, R. (1978) Teamwork in Theory and Practice. In R. Dingwall and J. McIntosh (eds) *Readings in the Sociology of Nursing*. Edinburgh: Churchill Livingstone.

McKnight, J. (1977) Professionalised Service and Disabling Health. In I. Illich, I. Zola, J. McKnight, J. Caplan, and H. Shaiken (eds) *Disabling Professions*. London: Marion Boyars.

McTernan, E. J. (1976) The Physician's Assistant. A Controversial Topic at Home and Abroad. *Medical Journal of Australia* **ii**: 760–63.

Mechanic, D. (1968) General Medical Practice in England and Wales. Its Organization and Future. *New England Journal of Medicine* **279**: 680–88.

— (1974) Factors Affecting Receptivity to Innovations in Health Care Delivery among Primary Care Physicians. In D. Mechanic (ed.) *Politics, Medicine and Social Science*. New York: John Wiley and Sons.

Medical Defence Union (1970). *Annual Report*.

Medical Practitioners Union (1980) *Medical Manpower and Career Structure*. An MPU Policy Document.

Mercer, G. (1979) *The Employment of Nurses*. London: Croom Helm.

Miller, D. S. and Backett, E. M. (1980) A New Member of the Team?

Extending the Role of the Nurse in British Primary Care. *Lancet* **ii**: 358–61.

Moore, M. F., Barber, J. H., Robinson, E. T., and Taylor, T. R. (1973) First Contact Decisions in General Practice – A Comparison Between a Nurse and Three General Practitioners. *Lancet* **i**: 817–19.

Moran, Lord (1958) Royal Commission on Doctors' and Dentists' Remuneration. Lord Moran's Evidence. *British Medical Journal* Supplement 1: 27–30.

Morrell, D. C. and Nicholson, S. (1974) Measuring the Results of Changes in the Method of Delivering Primary Medical Care – A Cautionary Tale. *Journal of the Royal College of General Practitioners* **24**: 111–18.

Mourin, K. (1980) The Role of the Practice Nurse and A Practice Nurse's Course: Content and Evaluation. *Journal of the Royal College of General Practitioners* **30**: 75–7; 78–84.

National Opinion Polls Ltd (1966) *Attitudes to Nurses.* (Unpublished.)

Navarro, V. (1978) *Class Struggle, the State and Medicine.* London: Martin Robertson.

Nelson, E. C., Jacobs, A. R., and Johnson, K. G. (1974) Patients' Acceptance of Physician's Assistants. *Journal of the American Medical Association* **228**: 63–67.

Newman, C. (1957) *The Evolution of Medical Education in the Nineteenth Century.* London: Oxford University Press.

Nightingale, F. (1859) *Notes on Nursing: What it is and what it is not.* London: Harrison and Sons.

Noack, H. (ed.) (1980) *Medical Education and Primary Health Care.* London: Croom Helm.

Nuffield Provincial Hospitals Trust (1960) *Casualty Services and their Setting.* London: Oxford University Press.

Nursing Mirror (1980) RCN Plans Appeal on Abortion Judgment. August 7: 5.

Parkhouse, J. (1979) The Development of Medical Manpower Forecasting and Modelling in Britain. In G. McLachlan, B. Stocking, and R. F. A. Shegog (eds) *Patterns for Uncertainty? Planning for the Greater Medical Profession.* Published for the Nuffield Provincial Hospitals Trust by Oxford University Press.

Parkhouse, J. and McLaughlin, C. (1976) Career Preferences of Doctors Graduating in 1974. *British Medical Journal* **ii**: 630–32.

Parkhouse, J. and Howard, M. (1978) A Follow Up of the Career

Preferences of Manchester and Sheffield Graduates of 1972 and 1973. *Journal of Medical Education* **12**: 377–81.

Pike, L. A. (1969) Health Education in General Practice. *Journal of the Royal College of General Practitioners* **17**: 133–34.

Pondy, L. R. (1970) *A Study of Patient Acceptance of the Physician's Assistant*. Duke University, Durham. (Unpublished.)

Queen's Institute of District Nursing (1970) *Nursing in the Community*. London: QIDN.

Radical Statistics Health Group (1977) *In Defence of the NHS*. London: RSHG.

Ratoff, L. (1973) More Social Work for General Practice. *Journal of the Royal College of General Practitioners* **23**: 736–42.

Reader, W. J. (1966) Professional Men. *The Rise of the Professional Classes in Nineteenth Century England*. London: Weidenfeld and Nicholson.

Redfern, S. J. (1979) *The Charge Nurse's Job Attitudes and Occupational Stability*. PhD Thesis, University of Aston. (Unpublished.)

Reed, D. E. and Roghmann, K. J. (1971) Acceptability of an Extended Nurse Role to Nurses and Physicians. *Medical Care* **9**: 372–77.

Reedy, B. L. E. C. (1972) The General Practice Nurse. *Update* **5**: 75–8; 187–93; 366–70; 433–38; 571–76.

— (1975) Telephone Messages Received by Seven General Practices. *Journal of the Royal College of General Practitioners* **25**: 916–23.

— (1977) The Health Team. In J. Fry (ed.) *Trends in General Practice 1977*. Published for the Royal College of General Practitioners by the British Medical Association.

— (1978) *The New Health Practitioners in America – A Comparative Study*. London: King Edward's Hospital Fund for London.

— (1979) Substitution and the Manpower Dilemma. In G. McLachlan, B. Stocking, and R. F. A. Shegog (eds) *Patterns for Uncertainty? Planning for the Greater Medical Profession*. Published for the Nuffield Provincial Hospitals Trust by Oxford University Press.

Reedy, B. L. E. C., Philips, P. R., and Newell, D. J. (1976) Nurses and Nursing in Primary Medical Care in England. *British Medical Journal* **ii**: 1304–306.

Reedy, B. L. E. C., Metcalfe, A. V., de Roumanie, M., and Newell, D. J. (1980a) The Social and Occupational Characteristics of

Attached and Employed Nurses in General Practice. *Journal of the Royal College of General Practitioners* **30**: 477–82.

— (1980b) A Comparison of the Activities and Opinions of Attached and Employed Nurses in General Practice. *Journal of the Royal College of General Practitioners* **30**: 483–89.

Reedy, B. L. E. C., Stewart, T. I., and Quick, J. B. (1980) Attachment of a Physician's Assistant to an English General Practice. *British Medical Journal* **281**: 664–66.

Reinkemeyer, M. H. (1966) *The Limited Impact of Basic University Programmes on Nursing: A British Case Study.* Manuscript of Dissertation from the University of California, Berkely. (Unpublished.)

Report of the Committee of the Central Health Services Council. General Practice Within the NHS (1954) (Cohen Report). London: HMSO.

Report of the Committee to Consider the Future Numbers of Medical Practitioners and the Appropriate Intake of Medical Schools (1957) (Willink Report). London: HMSO.

Report of the Committee on the Functions of the District General Hospital (1969) Central Health Services Council (Bonham Carter Report). London: HMSO.

Report of the Committee on Local Health Authority and Allied Personal Social Services (1968). London: HMSO.

Report of the Committee on Nursing (1972) (Briggs Report). London: HMSO.

Report of the Committee on Nursing Education (1964) (Platt Report). London: HMSO.

Report of the Committee on Senior Nursing Staff Structure (1966) (Salmon Report). London: HMSO.

Report on Consultants and Specialists (1948) (Spens Report). London: HMSO.

Report of the Interdepartmental Committee on Medical Schools (1944) (Goodenough Report). London: HMSO.

Report of the Joint Working Party on the Attachment of Nursing Services to General Practice (1970). London: HMSO.

Report of the Joint Working Party on the Medical Staffing Structure in the Hospital Service (1961) (Platt Report). London: HMSO.

Report of the Royal Commission on Medical Education (1968) (Todd Report). London: HMSO.

Report of the Royal Commission on the National Health Service (1979) (Merrison Report). London: HMSO.

Report on General Practitioners (1946) (Spens Report). London: HMSO.

Report of the Sub-Committee of the Standing Maternity and Midwifery Advisory Committee (1970). Domiciliary Midwifery and Maternity

Bed Needs (Peel Report). Central Health Services Council. London: HMSO.

Report of the Sub-Committee of the Standing Medical Advisory Committee (1963) The Field Work of the Family Doctor (Gillie Report). Central Health Services Council. London: HMSO.

Report of a Working Party on the Field of Work, Training and Recruitment of Health Visitors (1956). London: Ministry of Health.

Report of the Working Party on Management Structure in the Local Authority Nursing Services (1969) (Mayston Report). London: HMSO.

Reynolds, R. E. and Bice, T. W. (1971) Attitudes of Medical Interns Towards Patients and Health Professionals. *Journal of Health and Social Behaviour* **12**: 307–11.

Richardson, I. M., Howie, J. G. R., Durno, D., Gill, G., and Dingwall Fordyce, I. (1973) A Study of General Practitioner Consultations in North East Scotland. *Journal of the Royal College of General Practitioners* **23**: 132–42.

Riddick, F. A., Bryan, J. B., Gershenson, M. I., and Costello, A. C. (1971) Use of Allied Health Professionals in Internists' Offices. Current Practices and Physicians' Attitudes. *Archives of Internal Medicine* **127**: 924–31.

Robson, J. (1973) The NHS Company Inc? The Social Consequences of the Professional Dominance in the National Health Service. *International Journal of Health Services* **3**: 413–26.

Rosenthal, C. J., Marshall, V. W., Macpherson, A. S., and French, S. E. (1980) *Nurses, Patients and Families*. London: Croom Helm.

Rosenthal, H. (1980) *New Approaches to Health in the Community*. London Health Services Research Group.

Roy, R. R., Williams, C. B., and Bourns, H. K. (1973) Towards an Integrated Accident Service with Special Reference to Health Centres. *Update* **6**: 1345–350.

Royal College of General Practitioners (1968) The Practice Nurse. *Reports from General Practice* X.

— (1972) *The Future General Practitioner. Learning and Teaching*. London: British Medical Journal.

— (1973) Present State and Future Needs of General Practice. *Reports from General Practice* XVI.

Royal College of Nursing (1977) *Evidence to the Royal Commission on the National Health Service*. London: Royal College of Nursing.

— (1978) *The Duties and Position of the Nurse*. London: Royal College of Nursing.

— (1979) *The Extended Role of the Clinical Nurse*. London: Royal College of Nursing.

Royal College of Nursing and Royal College of General Practitioners (1974) *The Report of the Joint Working Party on Nursing in General Practice in the Reorganised NHS*. London: Royal College of Nursing.

Russell, M. A. H., Wilson, C., Taylor, C., and Baker, C. D. (1979) Effect of General Practitioners' Advice Against Smoking. *British Medical Journal* **ii**: 231–35.

Sadler, B. (1974) Legal Aspects. In D. M. Pitcairn and D. Flahault (eds) *The Medical Assistant*. World Health Organisation, Public Health Papers No. 60.

Sadler, A. M., Sadler, B. L., and Bliss, A. A. (1974) *The Physician's Assistant Today and Tomorrow*. Yale University Press.

Sagar, G., Morrow, T., and Lees, R. (1972) *Could you use a Physician's Assistant in your Practice? A Computer Analysis*. Queen's University, Ontario. (Unpublished.)

Scherer, K., Fortin, F., Spitzer, W. O., and Kergin, D. J. (1977) Nurse Practitioners in Primary Care. *Canadian Medical Association Journal* April 23: 856–62.

Scottish Home and Health Department. *Annual Reports*. 1960–1977.

Shepherd, M., Cooper, M., Brown, A. C., and Kalton, G. (1966) *Psychiatric Illness in General Practice*. London: Oxford University Press.

Shyrock, R. H. (1959) *The History of Nursing*. London: W. B. Saunders.

Sidel, V. W., Jefferys, M., and Mansfield, P. (1972) General Practice in the London Borough of Camden in 1968. *Journal of the Royal College of General Practitioners* **22**, Supplement No. 3.

Smith, R. A. (1974) Medex. In D. M. Pitcairn and D. Flahault (eds) *The Medical Assistant*. World Health Organisation, Public Health Papers No. 60.

Smith, J. W. and Mottram, E. M. (1967) Extended Use of Nursing Services in General Practice. *British Medical Journal* **iv**: 672–74.

Smith, J. W. and O'Donovan, J. B. (1970) The Practice Nurse – A New Look. *British Medical Journal* **iv**: 673–77.

Spector, R., McGrath, P., Alpert, J., Cohen, P., and Aikins, H. (1975) Medical Care by Nurses in an Internal Medical Clinic. Analysis of Quality and its Cost. *Journal of the American Medical Association* **232**: 1234–237.

Spitzer, W. O. and Kergin, D. J. (1973) Nurse Practitioners in Primary Care. *Canadian Medical Journal* **108**: 1005–16.

Spitzer, W. O., Sackett, D. L., Sibley, J. C., Roberts, R. S., Gent, M., Kergin, D. J., Hackett, B. C., and Olynich, A. (1974) The Burlington Randomised Trial of the Nurse Practitioner. *New*

England Journal of Medicine **290**: 251–56.

Stead, E. A. (1968) Educational Programs and Manpower. *Bulletin of the New York Academy of Medicine* **44**: 204–13.

Stimson, G. V. and Webb, B. (1975) *Going to see the Doctor.* London: Routledge and Kegan Paul.

Stimson, G. V. (1976) General Practitioners, 'Trouble' and Types of Patients. In M. Stacey (ed.) *The Sociology of the NHS.* Sociological Review Monograph No. 22.

— (1977) Social Care and the Role of the General Practitioner. *Social Science and Medicine* **11**: 485–90.

Storms, D. M. (1973) *Training for Nurse Practitioners: A Clinical and Statistical Analysis.* North Haven, Connecticut Health Services Research Series No. 4.

Stroller, R. J. and Geertsma, R. M. (1958) Measurement of Medical Students' Acceptance of Emotionally Ill Patients. *Journal of Medical Education* **33**: 585–90.

Swift, G. and MacDougall, I. A. (1964) The Family Doctor and the Family Nurse. *British Medical Journal* **i**: 1697–699.

Taylor, S. (1954) *Good General Practice.* London: Oxford University Press.

Tompkins, R. K. and Johnson, R. C. (1976) *Computer Based Paramedic Support and Audit.* Dartmouth-PROMIS Laboratory, New Hampshire. (Unpublished.)

Trafford, J. A. P., Ireland, R., McGonigle, M., Sharpstone, P., Halford Maw, L., and Evans, R. (1979) Screening for Hypertension: A Hospital Based Home Visiting Programme. *British Medical Journal* **ii**: 1556.

Tudor Hart, J. (1971) The Inverse Care Law. *Lancet* **i**: 405–12.

— (1976) General Practice Workload, Needs and Resources in the National Health Service. *Journal of the Royal College of General Practitioners* **26**: 885–92.

United States Department of Health, Education and Welfare (1977) *Research Digest Series. Nurse Practitioner Training and Deployment.* National Centre for Health Services Research.

Wadsworth, M. E. J., Butterfield, W. J. H., and Blaney, R. (1971) *Health and Sickness: The Choice of Treatment.* London: Tavistock Publications.

Wallace, C. M. (1975) Assessment of the Elderly. *Nursing Mirror* February 27: 54–60.

Wallace, B. B., Millward, D., Parsons, A. S., and Davies, R. H.

(1973) Unrestricted Access by General Practitioners to a Department of Diagnostic Radiology. *Journal of the Royal College of General Practitioners* **23**: 337–43.

Warin, J. F. (1968) General Practitioners and Nursing Staff: A Complete Attachment Scheme in Retrospect and Prospect. *British Medical Journal* **ii**: 41–5.

Warner, M. W. (1977) Family Medicine in a Consumer Age. *Canadian Family Physician* **23**: 31–4.

Waters, W. H. R., Sandeman, J. M., and Lunn, J. E. (1980) A Four Year Prospective Study of the Work of the Practice Nurse in the Treatment Room of a South Yorkshire Practice. *British Medical Journal* **280**: 87–9.

Weightman, G. (1978) When is a Nurse not a Nurse? *New Society* July 20: 130–32.

Weisz, F. H. (1972) *On Delegation in Medicine and Dentistry*. Samson Uityeverij. Alphen aanden Rijn-Brussel.

Wessex Regional Hospital Board (1964) *What do they really want?*

Whitfield, M. J. (1980) What do Consultants think of General Practice? *Journal of the Royal College of General Practitioners* **30**: 228–29.

Williams, W. O. (1970) A Study of General Practitioners' Workload in South Wales 1965–1966. *Journal of the Royal College of General Practitioners. Reports from General Practice* XII.

— (1977) The Receptionist – Barrier or Link? *Medical Secretary* **30**: 25–8.

Williamson, J. (1970) Preventive Aspects of Geriatric Medicine. *Modern Geriatrics* **1**: 24.

World Health Organisation (1975) *Fifth Report on the World Health Situation 1969–72*. Official Records of the World Health Organisation 225.

Wright, H. J. (1968) General Practice in South West England. *Journal of the Royal College of General Practitioners. Reports from General Practice* VIII.

Wrightson, M. (1975) Practice Nurses Get Together. *Nursing Mirror* January 2: 41–2.

Yankauer, A., Connelly, J. P., and Feldman, J. J. (1968) A Survey of Allied Health Worker Utilization in Pediatric Practice in Massachusetts and in the United States. *Pediatrics* **42**: 733–42.

Yeomans, R. E. (1977) Randomized Observations for Functional Analysis of Nurses in Expanded and Traditional Roles. *Military Medicine* **142**: 195–201.

NAME INDEX

SUBJECT INDEX

abortion 70
Acts: Apothecaries' *1815* 7–11; *1874* 12;
Health Insurance *1911* 15–18; Health
Services and Public Health *1968* 30;
Medical *1858* 8, 10–13, 15, 165;
Medical *1978* 47; Medicines *1978* 81;
Midwives' *1902* 34; National Health
Service *1946* 18–19, 35, 99; National
Health Service *1966* 67; *1974* 48;
Nurses' *1943* 99; Nurse Practice 71;
Nurses, Midwives and Health Visitors
1979 101; in 16th century 2–3, 33;
Reform *1832* 13; Registration of Nurses
1919 98, 100; Vocational Training *1977*
47
advantages of delegation 61–81, 121–23,
129, 146–55, 158
age: of doctors 51, 75–6, 119–20, 123–25,
152, 163; of nurses 157, 163; of
population 167–68
American Medical Association 85–6,
173; *see also* United States
American Nurses' Association 86–8, 100,
173, 177
ancillary staff 29–37, 112–13; and list size
56–7, 59; tasks of 77–81, 142–46; 157 *see
also* midwives; practitioners; nurses;
physician's assistants; receptionists;
secretaries; social workers
apothecaries 5–10; *see also* Society of
Apothecaries
Apothecaries' Act *1815* 7–11
Association for the Study of Medical
Education 21; *see also* medical
education
Association of General Practitioners 14;

see also Royal College of General
Practitioners
attachment 30, 33–7, 74, 122, 139; Report
on 81, 184; *see also* ancillary staff
autonomy *see* independence

Bills: Nurses' *1943* 99; Reform *1832* 13
Briggs Report *1972* 36, 94, 101–03, 184
British Medical Association 14, 16, 20,
22, 24, 34, 39, 53, 81, 174
British Nursing Association 97; *see also*
Royal College of Nursing

Camden 24–5
Canada: nurse practitioners in 82, 86,
149; physician's assistants in 90, 149;
studies in 62, 64, 138
Canadian Nurses' Association 86, 88, 175
capitation system 19–20, 23, 117 *see also*
fees
caring, as nurses' role 88, 103, 148–49,
158, 168
Central African Republic 83
Central Nursing, Midwifery and Health
Visiting Council 101
Charter for Family Doctor Service 22
chemists as prescribers 135
China 83
class differences 42, 65, 75, 107, 167
clinics 126, 155–56
Cohen Report *1954* 39, 184
Colleges *see* Royal College
community care 45–6, 166–68
Confederation of Hospital Service
Employees 107
Consultants and Specialists Report *see*
Spens Report